Me and Ms N

Me & Ms Menopause

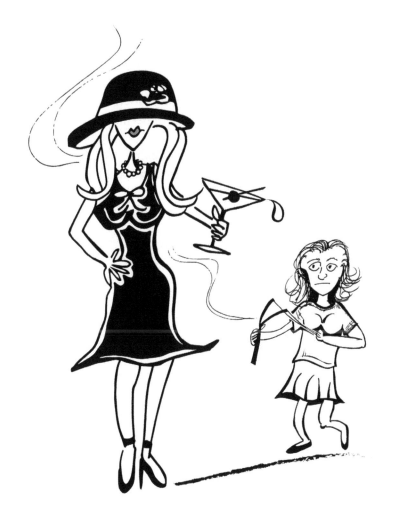

Jenni Townsend

Studio 554 Presents

Me and Ms Menopause

Copyright © 2015 Jenni Townsend

Cover illustration © 2015 Rachel Aitken
www.pipsqueakportfolio.com.au

Printed and bound in Australia by BookPOD

A Catalogue-in-Publication is available from the National Library of Australia.

ISBN: 978-0-646-94947-5

For the daughter

In memory of my mum and sister
and all the generations of women of
the past

And in the hope this book helps all
the women of the future with their
meeting with Ms Menopause.

Contents

INTRODUCTION 9

1. I YAM WHAT I YAM: THIS IS WHO I WAS............................13
2. YOU'RE TELLING ME HOW I FEEL?...................................17
3. THE FUNNY SIDE OF MS MENOPAUSE...............................27
4. MEET MS MENOPAUSE AND HER TROOPS, AKA SYMPTOMS 29
5. HISTORY OF MS MENOPAUSE..35
6. MS MEOPAUSE KNOCKS AT MY DOOR...............................40
7. CENTRELINK...OH DEAR!...51
8. HRT, OH GOODY! NOT!..55
9. DRUGS, DRUGS & MORE BLOODY DRUGS..........................59
10. MY LITTLE BLACK BOOK DEPRESSION & SUICIDE 63
11. AND OTHER THINGS..71
12. OH, OKAAY!...76
13. DOCTORS, AND ONE YIKES 79
14. SICKO 82
15. STOP PRESS! HELLO ADRENAL GLANDS 88
16. COINCIDENCE OR GUIDANCE?...97
17. Q&A 102
18. HELLO AND HAPPY NEW YEAR 2013!................................109
19. THESE DAYS TURNED OUT NOTHING LIKE I HAD PLANNED...118
20. NATURAL PROGESTERONE..125
21. DEAR PRIME MINISTER 131
22. HEALTHY VS UNHEALTHY..136
23. GOOD NEWS, CLARITY AND THE ARRIVAL OF "THE WHO FROM WHOVILLE"...140
24. HAPPY ST VALENTINES DAY..146

25. A QUICK BREATHER 149
26. A VERY SAD DAY 150
27. ANOTHER LETTER AND JEAN HAILES...................153
28. THE FIRST ALLERGIST...164
29. DEPRESSION AND SUICIDE... AGAIN 169
30. THE PSYCHIATRIST 173
31. THE ENDOCRINOLOGIST 177
32. IT NEVER RAINS BUT IT POURS 183
33. MY SHINY AND NEW ALLERGIST 190
34. CENTRELINK AGAIN! WITH A HAPPY ENDING...........193
35. BACK TO THE SPECIALISTS...................................197
36. VITAMIN D AND COLLAGEN...................................212
37. AND AN "I AM DISGUSTED"...................................220
38. BACTERIA IN THE GUT 224
39. THE LOGIC OF MS MENOPAUSE 228
40. THE MENOPAUSE CONSPIRACY 235
41. HAPPY NEW YEAR IT IS NOW 2014.........................257
42. AND ONWARDS WE GO—FEK!...............................291
43. WALKING, CREEPS AND DOGS 297
44. UPDATE ON INSURANCE COMPANIES, AND ONWARDS…..........300
45. HAPPY NEW YEAR 2015! 308
46. INSURANCE ZZZZZZZ 312
47. FEBRUARY 2015 ONWARDS...................................323
48. THE HORMONES OF A TWENTY-ONE-YEAR-OLD 342
49. TO BE FOREWARNED IS TO BE FOREARMED AKA THE
    HANDBOOK 353
50. MALE MENOPAUSE IN HONOUR OF ALL THOSE GREAT MEN ..377
51. THANK YOUS AND ONE "OH HELLO!".......................379

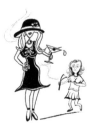

INTRODUCTION

I am gobsmacked that I was not more educated on the meeting I was to have with Ms Menopause. All I really thought this girl needed to know in regard to this encounter was:

- that it was inevitable
- that my mum met Ms Menopause in her fifties
- that we were finally free of periods
- that we didn't have to depend on birth control anymore
- that I was to leave my family for six months to handle the odd mood swing
- when it was over I would come back home and they would all still love me unconditionally.

Yay! A walk in the park, rock on into the rest of the chapters of my life disgracefully. Easy eh? Right? Yeahnah!

This book is my own personal experience and what I have learnt since my clash with Ms Menopause began. Daily I do battle with her, physically, emotionally and mentally.

I was completely baffled as to why women were not talking about Ms Menopause. Why has she been allowed to attack us in such a silent and hidden way? Only when she started to get really personal with me did I understand. It is not easy for women to talk about many of the things Ms Menopause has done to us, but I am going to talk about it. It is so very wrong that grandmothers, daughters, sisters, aunties, nieces, mothers, girlfriends, wives and best friends are dealing with this on their own. Every woman needs support and to be able to talk about it without being made to feel it is just something we go through so "soldier on ladies."

I was also completely bewildered by the generations of women of the past who had encountered Ms Menopause but didn't consider to forewarn following generations. My mum met Ms Menopause in her fifties, and that's it, just a memory I have. After the limited research I have done though, I feel very saddened by what those previous generations had to endure.

It is time to put Ms Menopause under the spot light and talk about her. I need to know that when my daughter meets with Ms Menopause, she will not be ambushed by the encounter or stripped of her life or who she is. I hope this book gives you a head start to help you to get through it, leaving you and your life intact.

But beware. Ms Menopause can plonk herself down in your home and stay for the rest of your lifetime. Yep! If things don't go well, she will not only go after the "ovary keepers", she will also affect your relationships, your family dynamics, your finances and your social life. A menopausal woman's ripple effect can be gigantic.

Men and women, you need to support and be there for your women, you won't think it is just something they go through when your sex life is suddenly non-existent, and your women are fully aware of how this is affecting their relationships, but they just can't seem to be who they were at this time in their lives. You won't think it's something women just go through when you are both in bed in the middle of a freezing winter, and your woman needs to sleep with the window wide open, and blankets kicked off because she is burning up from the inside out.

And these two examples are only the tip of the iceberg when it comes to Ms Menopause. She will pop up and affect parts of a menopausal woman's body that you didn't even know existed. Ms Menopause is cunning. Her effect on you, unless you have the right information, will be waved away as nothing to do with her, whilst she is standing in the dark shadows sniggering.

You will not think it is just something we have to deal with when Ms Menopause knocks and the woman in your life starts to show signs of depression. It won't matter how healthy, strong, funny, independent or happy that woman has been throughout her life, the depression can be a killer, literally. To women who are supporting women, pray Ms Menopause will not knock at your door for both of you at the same time. To women who deal with menopause in the same house at the same time, I say keep reading; hopefully I can help you all, even if it's in a small way.

I sit here and as I write I am really hoping that women all over the world are being supported by loved ones, but sadly I know that if I am doing it tough, women in other cultures will be doing it tougher. As for me, I have been and still am being supported by family and friends, but I still find this journey to be a lonely one. I also realize that it is not an easy journey for those supporting us. I thank God I have loved ones who are there for me, thank you all. It all would have been a hell of a lot harder and even more soul destroying without your love.

I have firstly and very selfishly, written this book for my daughter so that she is better prepared and will hopefully have a more gentle meeting with Ms Menopause.

Secondly, I am writing this in the hope it will help women to realise that they are not alone. I also believe that every woman has a right to deal with this stage of her life her own way. I hope it helps to finally put to bed those ideas that are being fed to us by the medical world such as the symptoms of Ms Menopause are exaggerated, and that you just have to suffer through it silently. We are menopausal women in the 21st Century; this is not the 1800s or 1900s. Why the hell is Ms Menopause still being allowed to bully us?

You know you!
You are intelligent women!
You know you are fighting to regain you!

I know who I was before Ms Menopause knocked on my door and I know who I am not anymore since her arrival.

Chapter 1

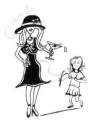

I YAM WHAT I YAM:
THIS IS WHO I WAS.

I started my work life at fifteen, working part time while still at school. I marched into my fulltime working life in 1980. I have worked, lived and played in Sydney, Melbourne, Perth, and Brisbane. Because Ms Menopause was so far in the distant future from me then, and due to the lack of education regarding her, I would more than likely have been asking "Who? What? Oh that! Whose shout?"

I gave birth to my beautiful daughter in 1992. I was thirty-one. I moved and settled in Brisbane where I still live today. My daughter has had quite a few health issues and operations on her foot and leg, but the girl is one month off being twenty-one as I write this and she's working and studying. Very proud of you my daughter.

I always worked except when family needed me. When my daughter was born I took a year off work to be with her. When I returned to the workforce I always held positions where I could balance motherhood as well as earning dollars. Family support played a huge role in my being able to do this. My mum passed over suddenly at sixty-seven years from a diabetic heart attack in 1995. Despite the pain, the grieving and the shock, we clawed our way back into life. I still miss her every day. I love you mum.

In 2004, with my daughter and best friend by my side, I cared for and lost my sister and my daughter's wonderful and favourite aunty to leukaemia. My beautiful sister passed over at her home, as she had wanted, a day after her forty-seventh birthday. My sister fought a very long, strong and courageous battle. She was all things feminine and beautiful, while I was the "ocker" climbing the trees. But the day she left, a very big piece of me left with her, and it was heartbreaking to see a parent, our dad, lose a child.

At the same time my daughter had to have an operation on the tendons in her foot, so it was quite a tag team from the children's hospital to the adult's hospital when the daughter and the sister were both still in care. The only positive was that the hospitals were right next to each other. A "chardy" or the occasional scotch plus a cry and a chat in between it all, also helped.

Almost straight after losing our sister to her horrible disease, our dad was diagnosed with bowel cancer. We again rallied, this time around this wonderful man, lovingly known as Pop. We all brought him home, as he wanted, and cared for him, but lost this special man in 2006. Again, through the grief, agony and pain we clawed and dragged ourselves back into life. I love you dad.

I had childhood asthma and always have been allergic to all sorts of bits and pieces like certain grasses, cats, housework, and so on. I am also allergic to penicillin. How did I find this fact out? Well, I was given a penicillin shot many years ago when I had the 'flu, which turned into a chest infection. I blew up with red welts all over my body. I then had to go and get another jab to counteract the penicillin. I needed two family members to come and get me, one to drive me home, the other to drive my car home.

I also had a reaction to a chemical I had dealt with in the workplace in 2007. I had tried to tell them it was not safe, but what do I know, I am just a girl! This chemical didn't just affect me, it also affected the girl I was working with. I went on and got it sorted though. Not once did these allergies stop me from living, earning my money, travelling and getting on with my life long-term.

I have had a few normal sick days off due to the 'flu etc, and yes even a few just because. Well you need a metal health day sometimes. In my younger days it was to go shopping or to get over a big night. Of course in my last job, where I was very happy, my days off were always legitimate sick days. As young Bart Simpson would say, "Didn't do it, wasn't there, you can't prove it."

I always stood up for the underdog, and bullying and outright rudeness always got my back up. I'm not saying I always got it right, I didn't. I am by no means perfect. I have held some really great positions in my working life, but felt comfortable and happy just being a pleb. I did pretty damn good in Ancient History at school and always loved this word 'pleb'. My interpretation of this word: The real workers!

One of my favourite things to do was dancing. Again, not saying I was good at it but must admit I was the best dancer and singer in the world after a number of slurpies, the adult ones with alcohol, and I always loved music.

I believe in kindness, but also believe kindness does not mean that you are a doormat that lets people walk all over you. I am not religious I am spiritual. It sounds like the "in thing" to say, but I am. I believe in God. I believe in Jesus. I am a great fan of the man. I believe at the end of our days we pass over and I believe in angels. Oh okay I will stop now. This is about Ms Menopause not the afterlife.

I kept working and settled into a position that I had decided, if I didn't get kicked out, was the job I was going to retire from. I was happy there. It was shift work and it suited my lifestyle and I loved the fact that my years of working with the public were over. I had always worked. In saying this though, women who stay at home to look after their families work just as hard and in my opinion, even harder at times. I chose to raise my daughter on my own. As much as work was a necessity, I always enjoyed working. Hey I am a Capricorn, it's what I do. I had planned to stay in the workforce until I was seventy years old. I even used to say, "You are going to have to crowbar my bony old fingers off the computer to get me out of here."

I was a strong, healthy, independent, oh and did I mention funny, woman who always put her family first. My life was settled and happy and I was content. I was multi-skilled in my place of work, happy to cover in different sections when and if needed, and I was at my happiest when I was really busy. Then, Ms Menopause knocked on my door.

I know now that she had been hanging around for a few years, but being unprepared, I didn't realize this until symptoms started to materialize. I also know now how Ms Menopause can strip you of who you once were and how she affects your health, family and loved ones, friendships, earning power, actually your whole life. Hey she can even give us girls a moustache that any man would be proud to have sitting under his nose!

Chapter 2

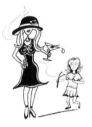

YOU'RE TELLING ME HOW I FEEL?

I find it interesting and totally annoying that the so-called experts have written quite a few articles telling me how I am feeling since Ms Menopause came and took over my life. Unless they have all encountered Ms Menopause themselves, they have no idea. After chatting with many women, there do not seem to be any mild or gentle or kind or nice symptoms, but the experts say there are. Every woman in the world who lives will meet Ms Menopause, whether they have had children or not, whether they have kept themselves healthy or not. As long as you have those girly bits, you are up for it!

I am not referring to those in the medical community, that comes later. No, I am talking about 'experts' who write books and articles on menopause which are often ignorant, flippant and sometimes downright stupid. What chance have women got to reach out for help, respect and support when this is the information offered? Now I do respect those who have studied and gained their qualifications and excelled in their chosen field, but I believe that life-experience can sometimes hold more weight than a certificate hanging on the wall. *And* I am sure that this chapter will be blamed on the rantings of a menopausal woman.

It also really annoys me that suddenly, every time a menopausal woman gets angry, it is now blamed on Ms Menopause. Am I defending her now? Yeahnah! I can get cranky because people just generally annoy me at times, as I do them.

The worst and saddest part of this is that many women now feel they haven't a voice anymore. Use your voices girls, as you always have. Unfortunately it won't always be the medical community or society making you feel you haven't a voice. Ms Menopause will at times grab you by the throat and turn you into a crying mess for no reason except for the fact that she can.

It's the same old same old even when I had a partner. One time he responded to me with this little beauty, "It's okay, it's just that time of month talking." Talking? I think I recall screaming. My response was, "It has nothing to do with "that time of month", YOU ANNOYED ME BY YOUR ACTIONS!" I wish I'd had the luxury to say to a partner whom I had annoyed, "Settle petal, don't worry, it is just your prostate talking." Sounds a bit unhinged, doesn't it. Well so does telling a woman she is angry only because of "that time of month," or because we girls are dealing with Ms Menopause. Please ladies, as hard as it will be at times, try and not allow anyone to take your voices away.

In a local newspaper a few weeks ago, there was a two-page spread on men's prostate problems. Very much needed I say, though it did make me ponder as to where the two-page spread on menopause was located. There was no spread on menopause. As I was flipping through other pages I came upon an article about depression written by a well-known doctor. He wrote about, well pretty much everything, except menopause. Ok yeah, I was baffled and annoyed but not at all surprised. So I sent off an email to him asking why he had made no mention of menopause in his writings on depression. I haven't heard back from him. He must be busy.

Today I opened the Sunday paper and there, in black and white, was a one and a quarter page spread on, da da da da, Menopause! Yay! I have to make mention that the other quarter of the pages were advertising "youth creams" and "youth serums" for women. Oh okay, so those creams give us back the oestrogen and progesterone we are losing, do they? Well we all know the answer to that! It didn't take long before I put the paper down to ponder what I was reading. Why does it seem, always, that there is an invisible blanket surrounding Ms Menopause and the truth? Ms Menopause takes the lives of many women around the world. There are those who will also say that Ms Menopause is not an illness. Well we women know that menopause is a part of our natural life, but Ms Menopause affects our bodies by squeezing and sucking those hormones out of our ovaries in a silent, stealthy way which means a lot of women are suffering illnesses in this phase of their lives which are not being associated with menopause. A lack of education and facts results in not knowing all our options. They try to blame a lot of these illnesses on old age. Hey, *wait a minute*, I am *middle*-aged! But these illnesses are affecting so many menopausal women as the medical community continues to sweep the truth under the rug. Geez must be pretty damn lumpy by now, how much can you sweep under a rug before people start noticing?

Well I didn't, I was totally clueless. Ms Menopause's job is simple: she arrives, she starts to drain most of your oestrogen, all of your progesterone and a little of the small amount of testosterone we girls have. Sounds easy, but the effect of losing these hormones can have a catastrophic effect on your body. For many, this is when unexpected illnesses may start appearing. But you know what? It shouldn't be like this and it doesn't have to be like this! So Ms Menopause is being *allowed* to become an illness for the menopausal woman. I rest my case your honour!

Now back to that Sunday paper spread. I want the experts to know I disagree with quite a lot of what you said.

Firstly Ms Professor, your comment that this can be the start of a new and positive life stage for women. Well I need to ask you, upon what facts do you base your "can be" when 75 to 80% of women worldwide suffer when it is time for Ms Menopause to come knocking? Have you even met her yet and experienced her wrath, even to a less harsh degree compared to other women? If so I am happy for you that you sit in that 20 to 25%, they say, of women that don't do so badly, or has she just not knocked for you yet? Again, what hope have women to reach out for help and support when women are not even supporting women?

I did, Professor, like your comment that older women have a lot to contribute. I already knew that, it was just good to see it in print, but I don't agree with your comment that it can be one of the best phases of a women's life. Here we see that "can be" again, sorry professor, you just didn't do it for me. I believe it "could be" if women were given all their options as well as all the correct information before their own journey even starts, but we all know that is not the case. Why?

Oh hello Gynaecologist, what a very important job you have. I must say straight up, that even though you are the expert on all the girly bits of a woman, I didn't come across anything, nada, zilch, stating that you are the expert on Ms Menopause. I did agree with your comment though, saying symptoms can start years before. I found this out too late, but did you know that a prolapsed vagina, and even a prolapsed bladder are also due to oestrogen deficiency caused by Ms Menopause? I thought that any prolapse of any kind in a woman was due to having too many kids or not doing pelvic exercises after giving birth. Nowhere ever in my past had I heard Ms Menopause being mentioned in regard to this.

I am sure you are thinking, who the hell do you think you are, maybe rightly so, but please can you explain these two symptoms to the numerous women who haven't had children? Yet these problems only pop up, or out, sorry, couldn't resist the pun, when Ms Menopause comes knocking. Here are some facts for you Gynaecologist, prolapsed bladders and vaginas are commonly associated with menopause. Prior to menopause womens' bodies create oestrogen, a hormone that helps to keep the muscles in and around the vagina strong. Both ovaries stop creating oestrogen if and when Ms Menopause is done, and those muscles then weaken.

You wrote a piece also on the truth about HRT, Hormone Replacement Treatment. Sorry but did I miss something or are you giving us the truth about HRT in a part two spread sometime in the future? It was good to see that you didn't even pretend to know anything about it though. Again, you could well be sitting there with your nose out of joint, but you know what? I don't care, I am writing this firstly for my daughter and all women who are made to feel, and who might be made to feel in the future, non-existent. What you think of me is irrelevant. Actually shame on both you and the Professor, you both work at a Women's Health Foundation, and this is the best you can do?

Now, before continuing, I have looked into a Womens' Health Centre and have discovered it is a medical clinic with all women doctors. What I want to know is do these clinics with all these women doctors have a few that also specialise in menopause? I have been told they give great support but how much does that cost? And I do know for a fact that women will have to pay more to go to these clinics and none of them bulk bill. I also noticed some women doctors charge a higher fee to see them. Why is this? I hope it is not a case where desperate women, struggling to survive through menopause, are seen as profit.

The cost for a menopausal woman to be treated safely and with respect is beyond many womens' means. It should not be only the rich menopausal woman who does not have to suffer. Even though I am happy that the rich menopausal woman does not have to suffer, every woman from all walks of life should be able to have affordable access to treatment and good information.

As for HRT, I do feel we are damned if we do and damned if we don't. Keep reading, I write some truths about HRT later. I did however agree with you that many women have been left untreated and suffer much more than they should. Maybe this is because they have tried to speak up about their problems but are not being listened to. You also didn't enlighten me one iota about Ms Menopause.

Hello Naturopath, you are the first and the one and only of the experts that actually excited me. I agree that just because a product is said to be natural, it doesn't mean it's ok. I am a little confused though, as to why you said the "cure" word in regard to menopause. In my research and speaking with other women, not once did we think that natural treatments and products would actually "cure" menopause. Being intelligent women, we thought perhaps they might help to alleviate some symptoms, but as I have stated previously, my research is very limited. I would love to know where the cure word is mentioned on products in regard to menopause.

You went on to speak about natural foods that may benefit woman so I will look at this later. I could have kissed you when you spoke about phytoestrogens, the natural hormone in foods, you did well Naturopath.

Hello Sex Educator. Well regardless of whether I think your writings were crap or not, okay then to be truthful, I thought your writings were pure crap, you win, because at the moment I am a single woman. Of course I still have quite a few things to say though. As I was reading your so-called expert advice, I found you to be entirely patronizing towards women. We women know now that our libido and our sex drive falls. Don't you think that every woman in a loving relationship would love to be able to perform? You said, "Women are just slower to get there, things may take longer. Touching and talking to each other will help, it's no longer 'wham bam thank you ma'am." Wow! Ok, first of all I feel very sorry for you that you think it has only ever been wham bam thank you ma'am. Secondly, it would concern me, considering you are a sex educator, that this is what you teach in the sessions you conduct with people. Yes the "wham bam thank you ma'am" has its place at times, even so, I would hate to be in one of your sessions and be given this "expert" advice. I am quite sure I would feel, if I didn't know any better, (but luckily I do) that there was something wrong with me if I wanted a little bit more and something a little bit slower than the "wham bam thank you ma'am".

From what you, the expert, also stated regarding the touching and talking, isn't that how a loving relationship is anyway, even if you are not going through menopause? As for it taking longer, it is a well-known fact that women have always taken longer to "get there". You then went on to say women have to take some responsibility for keeping sex and intimacy on the agenda, and you advised women to read some well written erotica to help get in the mood, then continued to tell women to wear something sexy that makes her feel flirty and comfortable, such as a lacy nightie that glides over bumps and stretch marks, geez all mighty, I can feel an outright roar of laughter bubbling to the surface, you are joking aren't you? This is the *best* advice you can give us? This sounds like advice from a 1950s magazine, laughable, stupid and totally outdated!

For women, menopause is not a time when we decided to say, "That's it! You are not getting it anymore. You have exhausted your quota for the rest of your natural life, now feck off!" It is a time when we women are losing our hormones dear! You are the expert and I had to remind you of this? The women I have spoken to know how it is affecting their healthy relationships. Your advice did nothing but make women feel bad at a time when they need support. Women, if this sex educator's suggestions help you, I say great! Enjoy! For all the other women out there who felt these comments made them feel bad and even a failure in that department, please don't take it on board. I know sex is important in a good relationship, but when you look at the amount of time you are in bed compared to the rest of your time with each other, well it just ain't that big guv! You still have your companionship, love, laughter, holding of hands, big cuddles, beautiful kisses, slothing over each other on the lounge watching a movie. Do not let a so-called sex educator make you feel less of a woman just because at this time in your life Ms Menopause is affecting your sex life.   Actually, take a moment and roughly calculate how many times you *have* done it! Yeah, that's right, and women can't be cut some slack at this time in their lives? Feckin unbelievable!

Hey Sex Educator, how do you get your certificate in this field anyway? You really don't want to know what is swirling around in my thoughts, and please excuse my ignorance, but I am thinking you should be calling yourself a Relationship Educator. As far as I'm concerned, *that* title could be debated as well.

Hello Psychologist. Firstly, thank you for taking on the role of helping people to lead happier and more meaningful lives. I also hear that you are an expert on human behaviour, but why are you talking to me about Ms Menopause when she is not a human behaviour? Ms Menopause does cause different behaviour in all women as a result of the loss of hormones. Also all the different symptoms we all of a sudden have thrown at us cause changes of behaviours, so in my small world, your comments were, once again, of no real help. Let's get into it, shall we?

For a start, you went on to say that menopause does not cause depression, "as such." Three words for you, Yes It Does! This is a very dangerous and misguided statement. Here is a fact for you: during this time in women's' lives, they are three times more likely than the general population to be diagnosed with depression and they are more likely to commit suicide than at other times in their lives.

Psychologist, what do you mean by, "as such?" I am confused. "Menopause does not cause depression as such." So what the hell does that mean? You go on and tell us why we feel sad. You say it forces women to realise the aging process is starting. Other experts, at times, have also swept it away with statements about the empty nest syndrome. So this is what I reckon, because as we all know, I am a great expert on me. Firstly you said "forces". I've never felt forced to look my aging process in the face. If anything I want to get old, but I want to be me and healthy throughout it. I also get that aging is a part of life. What? Do you think we women don't know that? Hey, did you know that only a few generations ago women were not living long due to Ms Menopause, but prior generations of women were living a very long time? Why is that? Ok, back to the subject at hand about your "aging" mumbo jumbo.

I was ready to embrace Ms Menopause, hell yeah, I was even going to throw a menopause party to celebrate her arrival. Well that hasn't happened. You know, I haven't got any issues with moving into the last chapters of my life. What I do have a problem with is all the ill-informed, ignorant, and stupid comments, you "experts" dribble on about to us women who are trying and struggling to survive during this time.

Now the empty nest syndrome is interesting. Try throwing that one out to the woman who is sobbing in the arms of her partner because her heart is ripped out because of not being able to have a baby, or to the woman who has chosen not to have children. It's her body and her right, but both their meetings with Ms Menopause are just the same as a woman who has borne a child.

As for my thoughts on the empty nest syndrome, of course it's natural to miss our young adult children when they fly the nest. At times you even get to see your child leave the nest a few times so that it actually becomes like water off a duck's back, but what a blessing and joy to see your child take their rightful place in the world.

I agree that exercise can help. You suggested that ways of improving our mood could be by "finding a sense of achievement, satisfaction". You again suggested "reading a good book, cooking a beautiful meal or closing a business deal". Lucky the business deal bit was tossed in, otherwise I also would have thought your words were from a 1950s magazine, outdated and stupid. You went on to say, "find things that give you a sense of reward". Okay then, well my sense of reward would be to be who this missy was before Ms Menopause knocked on my door, just older, wiser and more mature. Well ok the mature bit is debatable. Your comments really give me a sense of, well they sound condescending to me. I am only fifty-one, I am not ready to be put out to pasture just yet, regardless of what all you experts think.

Finally, yes there is more, you stated earlier that in a girl's life we experience anxiety and depression at two to three times the rate of men. I get that as we have periods, and we have those hormones, no-brainer there Psychologist. Then you went on to say that by middle-life, this disparity reduces. Oh, okay. I am not going to repeat myself on this one, but what does disparity mean? I'm assuming you are saying that our anxiety and depression disperses and levels out. What a crock of crap!

Okay I am going to have to repeat myself here. Dealing with menopause-induced depression is a very real thing, and I won't allow you to tell me it isn't because I am living it. Again, your comments, like the rest in the spread, have done absolutely nothing to help menopausal women. Me still thinketh Ms Menopause is too big, or is it that it would cost too much money, to ensure that women are treated with respect in all stages of their lives? It is women's right to be treated with respect for who they are and all they have done. A woman has the right to live her life in exactly the way that suits her, in a state of health and happiness for the rest of her natural life.

Ok, I have now responded to all the experts in that spread. All I really got out of all that was: CAN BE THE TRUTH CURE AS SUCH, SO WHAM BAM THANKYOU MA'AM! Hey, this could be a book title! Except for Naturopath, whose only really curious word was "cure," I got nothing out of that. Sometimes it sounded like you were making it up as you went, mostly pure rubbish. My friend who spoke to me about it actually found it really embarrassing.

Unless you all come up with facts and insight, and can offer real help for a menopausal woman to find her way back to herself safely, I don't want you to speak on my behalf ever again about what I am going through.

Your flippant attitude and ignorant remarks are not only embarrassing and disrespectful to women, they are also dangerous for the menopausal woman. Pull your heads in and stop thinking that we women are going to continue to believe and accept everything and anything you tell us about Ms Menopause. It is unbelievable that we are in the 21st Century and you lot are still trying to deal with women as if we are living in the past. Maybe you all need to update your textbooks, that is if there is even a mention of menopause in them!

Chapter 3

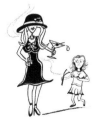

THE FUNNY SIDE OF
MS MENOPAUSE

Umm. Oh sorry, I am still thinking about it... la la la. Oh okay! I have heard from a few people that the stage production *Menopause* is hilarious.

Look, all joking aside, I love laughter. I can't wait until once again I have one of those laughs that bubble up from the core of my stomach and makes my head tilt back, my face towards heaven, and the roar of laughter comes out, loud and damn proud! Within my family and friends, we have had a few giggles. Hey, I nearly got a giggle out of some of the comments from the experts. I also hope you get a giggle from time to time while reading your way through all the seriousness of this subject.

I love laughter as much as I love music, both are fantastic for the soul. However throughout my dealings with Ms Menopause and the way in which my family, my friendships, in fact my whole life has been affected, I'm sorry, I can't seem to find her funny side right now.

Chapter 4

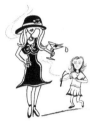

MEET MS MENOPAUSE AND HER TROOPS, AKA SYMPTOMS

The following is from a website I found. I could not have said it better myself:

> Menopause symptoms can be psychological physical, emotional, or cognitive. Some of the symptoms are easier to live with than others. Severity can range anywhere from mild to completely disruptive and debilitating. Many of the symptoms are often difficult to live with as they interfere in relationships and a woman's ability to function and cope in the world.
>
> The body goes through changes that can affect a woman's social life, a woman's feelings about herself and her ability to function at work.
>
> Hormones have a profound impact on the brain which can result in a variety of menopause symptoms that appear to be a psychological disturbance. The inability to cope in life can be completely overwhelming. Many women report it feels as if they will lose their minds.

In society and even in the medical world, there can sometimes be a flippant attitude that simply dismisses a woman's suffering as insignificant because "you are just menopausal." My doctor who has travelled with me on my journey with Ms Menopause has been great. I believe he and I were both learning at the same time, but as time has passed, he seems to have become more knowledgeable. Many doctors however, have very limited knowledge of how to deal with and treat the menopausal woman, or have the attitude of "we are just menopausal and it is something we just have to go through."

I was totally ignorant of how horrible and terrible Ms Menopause can be to women. I thought there were only two symptoms that we might have to deal with: hot flushes and mood swings. This is backed up by the fact that these are the only two symptoms mentioned on a regular basis if a piece is written on Ms Menopause. Let's meet Ms Menopause's troops:

- Period irregularities, excessive bleeding, on-and-off bleeding, decreased bleeding, bleeding that lasts longer than my last relationship, cravings for sweets, gall bladder pain, excessive fatigue, memory loss, heart palpitations, anxiety, weight gain, headaches, migraines, mood swings, loss of sexual drive, depression, irritability, dry skin, breast pain, vaginal dryness, hair loss, fibroids, incontinence, joint pain, joint stiffness, inability to deal with stress, sleep disturbance, difficulty concentrating, mental confusion, disorientation, dizziness, feeling of dread, apprehension or doom, night sweats... I need to take a breath!... inability to cope, increase in allergies, bloating, exacerbation of symptoms of an existing health condition or illness, hair growth, fatty tissue in the stomach, hot flushes, nausea, weakness of the immune system, sadness, insomnia, body chills, body odour changes, internal shaking or tremor-like feeling, pain during sex, itching skin or feeling of ants crawling under your skin, panic attacks, urinary infections, brittle nails, burning tongue, electric shocks, digestive problems, brain fog, gum problems and muscle tension. Try saying all that in one breath, you will be blue, crashing to the ground in no time!

I discovered these symptoms after talking to other women and doing some research. Menopause also can cause the following: heart disease, breast cancer, ovarian cancer, diabetes, osteoporosis, endometrial cancer, thyroid problems, prolapsed vagina and prolapsed bladder.

I am sure there are those of you in the medical profession who are reading this, who are right now saying, "humbug, nonsense." But let me tell you about the troops that have personally attacked me: period irregularities, excessive fatigue, cravings for sweets, memory problems, heart palpitations (these are fun, like your chest is going to burst with every beat of your heart), anxiety (I dealt with this when I lost loved ones, but still was able to crawl and then march back into life and work), headaches, weight gain, mood swings, depression, irritability, breast pain, dry skin, joint pain, inability to deal with stress, sleep disturbance, difficulty concentrating, mental confusion and disorientation, feeling of dread, dizziness, (I can't start cleaning the fridge out as every time I bend down and come up I get dizzy, gee sorry family. At times I can be upright and feel dizzy. I just stand still waiting to see if it lands me on the ground), inability to cope, (this one makes me feel crazy), increase in allergies, exacerbation of existing health conditions and illnesses, bloating, (I have been so bloated in my stomach that I swear blind I do the pregnancy waddle! For those of you who have been pregnant, I use my stomach as a resting place for my arms again), nausea, weakness of the immune system, sadness, insomnia (I was sleeping two hours at a time, if I slept for four hours I thought I was doing well, up and down all night, sleep, when it came, was often at inappropriate times. Now to contradict what I have just said, at the peak of my depression I was sleeping all day, go figure, no wonder we feel we are going crazy), internal shaking or tremor-like feelings, and body chills, (I used to start work at 6am. In winter it is freezing. All the guys and I used to turn up to start our shifts in at least two or three jumpers. By maybe 9am, they had all pretty well stripped down to just their uniforms. Not me! I was still working with all my coverings on, chilled to the bone), feeling of ants crawling under my skin, electric shocks, (a weird one and even weirder to explain), muscle tension and brain fog.

Also, I have just been advised by my doctor that I have the beginnings of a prolapsed bladder. He then told me it was due to being oestrogen deficient because of menopause. I was in shock and I was angry, not because of the diagnosis as it can be fixed with exercise. Actually as I am typing I am doing my exercises. Just watch out for the prolapse. If you don't get it looked at, it can end up popping out like a coin bag. Serious. Just sayin'—that's what I've been told. I was annoyed that Ms Menopause was able to rear her head in another part of my body without me being aware that this can happen.

Here are some facts about a few symptoms. I don't know how old these reports are, I get tired just writing, so my research is probably considered very limited and ignorant to the experts, I have no illusions that I know everything about Ms Menopause. What I will say though, with great confidence, is that I am an expert on my body and how I am affected. I am my own waddling, talking, breathing and crying expert.

- **Menopause, Depression and Suicide:** Chemical imbalances brought on by menopause lead to women becoming clinically depressed. If the depression continues, suicide becomes a genuine risk factor for the woman who is then suffering from menopause-induced depression.

  According to the World Health Organization, suicide rates among women increase with age and peak at menopause. Middle-aged women are committing suicide. Another study from America reported a 49% increase in suicide or suicide attempts for a woman over fifty due to hormonal changes. Menopause is a risk factor for depression. During menopause, women are three times more likely than the general population to be diagnosed with depression. Women during menopause are more likely to commit suicide than at other times in their lives.

When I mentioned the above report to a member in the medical community I was advised that that study concerns only women who live in America. What? And your point is? You think American ovaries are different to Aussie ovaries? And let's not forget that there would be many multi-cultural ovaries living in America as well.

- **Menopause and Alzheimer's Disease:** 70% of Alzheimer's Disease sufferers are women. A study suggests that the increased incidence of Alzheimer's Disease in women who are older could be due to the oestrogen deficiency and that ERT - oestrogen replacement therapy- may be useful for preventing or even delaying the onset of dementia.

- **Menopause and Chronic Inflammation (CI):** Hormonal changes in menopause causes CI that has already, or will lead to, more debilitating diseases. It is well documented that symptoms of CI do increase during and after menopause and is linked to heart disease, cancer, diabetes and depression. The root and core of chronic inflammation is an imbalanced immune system. The hormone system is very much interwoven with the immune system.

- **Menopause and Diabetes:** During Menopause, hormone changes cause fluctuations in blood sugar levels. A study showed that while we are dealing with sleep disorders and insomnia, they can make our blood sugar levels rise. Weight gain that can occur during menopause affects the blood sugar levels, which cause the onset of diabetes. A study done over four years researching post-menopausal women showed that even though none of these women had diabetes prior to Ms Menopause knocking, a number of women had become diabetic. The results showed diabetes and menopause are linked.

I have to take a moment here. Dear God, please keep me healthy in this debilitating journey Ms Menopause is taking me on. If I can't get her out of my door in my lifetime, please help me to be stronger than her. Thank you God.

Now I am sure you all may think it is strange that I have prayed to stay healthy, even with all I am already dealing with. Well, I pray that I don't get cancer, that I don't commit suicide, that I don't get Alzheimer's or diabetes or any other debilitating or life threatening illness. I don't want to die because of Ms Menopause as a lot of women are. As I mentioned, my mum died suddenly of a diabetic heart attack at sixty-seven with no prior history of diabetes until being diagnosed with "old-age" diabetes.

I now wonder, did we lose this wonderful woman too early? My wish is that generations to come will not lose their beautiful women or themselves too early or unnecessarily

Chapter 5

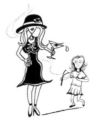

HISTORY OF MS MENOPAUSE

Prior to the last 100 years or so, as most women entered menopause it meant the end of their expectant natural life. If a woman did live through it, they were considered to have outlived their usefulness and were considered a less valued member of society. I have gone back as far as my limited research has allowed:

- **1600s:** Women who were menopausal were judged as being witches and thrown in the river to drown. Imagine if I had lived in this time! It would have been into the river with me because I'm going through "the change." With one last breath left, they would have dragged me out of that bloody river and then tossed me back in because… I believe in angels. Again on my last breath, I would have been dragged out then tossed back in due to my big mouth and my opinions. At the end of it all they would have dragged me out, dried me off and burnt me at the stake!
- **1700s:** Didn't find much about this century, I am sure it was just as barbaric as the 1600s.

- **1800s:** In my research I read somewhere that a woman did a study on women who in the mid 1800s were being admitted to insane asylums. Women were being put away due to the fact that they were going through menopause. This study showed, after researching these women's' admittance forms, that the reason given on many of these forms was "lunacy". So their men were getting them put away, marrying younger women and moving on with their lives. Well not much has changed except nowadays those men would be buying a red sports car to go with the younger woman.

Men in the1800s were doing unspeakable and terrible things to their women who were going through menopause. It was very much out in the open, it was scary and terribly sad. Dr Louise Fox Croft, a specialist in medical history, wrote, "Hot Flushes Cold Science: A History of the Modern Menopause." The following quotes an article in the Daily Mail Online on her book.

> There was a physician, Edward Tilt, who was quite popular for women who were suffering with menopause. In this generation they thought there was a direct link between the womb and the brain, which predisposed women to insanity. The remedy, they concluded, was straightforward - such women should be locked up. It was in this century menopause began being viewed as a disease, this then lead to bizarre treatments and extremely dangerous surgeries. It was decided that a woman's ovaries were the basis of a woman's essence and all she was, sprang from them. Should the ovaries become "diseased" ie cease to function in menopause then all hell could break loose! It was decided that the ovaries needed to be surgically taken out. It would make a woman more biddable, cleaner in mind and body and more industrious. The surgical removal of the ovaries was used excessively in attempts to "cure" mental disorders, sex drive and hysteria. In the 1800s women were supposed to only want to be motherly.

> Out of 200 surgical removals of the ovaries, eighty-nine women died. They managed to reduce the rate of mortality over the next two decades due to the introduction of anaesthesia.

The surgeon maintained he was performing these surgeries to alleviate the suffering of women but some of his colleagues believed the only people who benefited, financially and professionally, were the surgeons.

So any talk of sex and off with her ovaries! This would make the woman spiral faster into menopause as all her progesterone and oestrogen would be gone in one fell swoop. And note that for a time women were having their ovaries ripped out without anaesthesia!

Another bloke, Isaac Baker Brown, insisted insanity resulted from excessive desire. Umm I think that's called a woman's sex drive, mate, and it's normal. Let us not forget at this time in history, even if a woman thought about sex it was considered excessive. Well this butcher recommended clitoridectomy, the surgical removal of the clitoris. It was claimed by them that removing our clitoris it would stop hysteria, idiocy, mania and even death.

It goes on to tell a story about a women going through menopause who had sadly attempted to commit suicide. The husband had her put into an asylum, her symptoms got worse, so in came Isaac Baker Brown who performed, you guessed it, a clitoridectomy on this woman. A week later he reckons she was sleeping better, but she wouldn't own up to feeling better and complained of her skin being dry and burning hot. Isaac Baker Brown "begged to differ." He ignored her hot flushes and recorded that she "merely, at times perspired freely".

These poor women were in the hands of mad men who just did whatever they wanted with these women. The Medical Society of today is still telling woman rubbish about how they are feeling. You know, I do "get" why many women suffered in silence. I would too if it meant I would get to keep all my girly bits!

By the end of the century, they were starting to realize that a woman's sex hormones might be involved.

- **1900s:** Things were starting to change. It was thought a woman's suffering might be relieved by hormone treatment, but still, men had their own way of speaking. In 1966, Robert Wilson said that a menopausal woman's body was a "galloping catastrophe" - I have to agree - "which only oestrogen could repair. Thus, this will make a woman much more pleasant to live and deal with, not dull and unattractive."

  Interestingly enough though, as he was going on about hormone replacement, it turns out that he was being funded by a pharmaceutical firm whose profits from HRT took off over the next thirty years. Robert even placed an advertisement in the journal of The American Medical Association in 1975 that claimed, "Almost any tranquilizer used might calm her down, but at her age, oestrogen might be what she really needs."

  Adverts like his really helped the sale of HRT, but it came at a cost. His wife, who had taken HRT, died from breast cancer in 1988. This woman kept her illness a secret to protect the reputation of her husband, Robert Wilson. This was made public by his son, so did Robert Wilson know of his wife's suffering but choose to also protect his reputation? Maybe not, I just find it curious that it was made public by the son and not by the husband himself. We will get back to Louise's piece a bit later. In 1970 there was a British doctor who apparently was using electric shock therapy to treat/cure menopause.

- **21st Century:** Louise ends her piece with, "Even today, secrecy surrounds menopause. Women are reluctant to talk about it, some men are embarrassed by it, but to really understand it women need to speak up. The experience a woman has with menopause needs to be and has to be recorded, published and - not least - believed." Thank you again Louise Fox Croft.

- **2016:** Boo! Well here we are today and what have I learnt? That compared to generations past, we women are safer in the respect that some butcher is not going to come along and hack out our ovaries and clits willy-nilly, and that we are not going to be drowned in rivers or admitted to mental asylums as easily as they were in the past. But in saying that, we are not safer in regard to HRT or those flippant attitudes of the medical world or society itself.

So to sum up, same old crap. The disrespect and the still obvious disregard for menopausal women is just done in a more subtle, quieter way now. HRT and Ms Menopause herself is still killing women. We are still are not being listened to, or being taken seriously when we try and speak up about Ms Menopause.

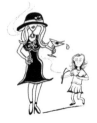

Chapter 6

MS MEOPAUSE KNOCKS AT MY DOOR

A s we now know, Ms Menopause is in your life for years before she actually knocks. I think about this now. My periods were always regular and on time. I do recall a time prior to 2010 when I had some irregularities with my periods, but by the time I had decided to get it checked out they resumed to their normal and steady cycle. Beware of the saying "stress can affect your period," yes it can, but knowing what I know now and the age I was, I would have ensured I went to the doctor to check if Ms Menopause was on the horizon. Irregular periods could be something else as well so let us not give Ms Menopause all the credit.

I just need to mention that in 1998, we brought a puppy for my daughter who had just started grade one at school. I started to get rashes, and blood tests confirmed I was allergic to the dog. When I told my then six year old daughter, "Okay daughter, it's either the dog or me," her response was, "See you mum." Yes the offbeat humour starts at a very early age in our family. Off I went to the allergist to have a year of desensitization needles. I was still working and life went on as usual around these needles, except when family needed me.

In 2010 I started to get rashes on my skin again and I wasn't sleeping properly. A few of us would gather at work and discuss my rash. I remember saying, "I can live with the rash," but before I could finish my sentence, a mate said "but it's the lack of sleep which is the killer." All I could say was, "Yeah!" If I knew what I know now, I would have questioned her a bit more on that comment. Obviously she was having sleeping problems too.

In October 2010 I went to my doctor and had blood tests done. I was forty-three "something-or-others" into menopause, you know I am still not too sure what that means. I started taking herbal tablets that are said to help with menopause. My doctor did explain that before Ms Menopause shows herself by stopping our periods, our hormones have been up and down like a roller coaster for a few years already. My allergy rate was up as well so I booked an appointment with the allergist I had seen in 1999, but I couldn't see him until August 2011.

Unfortunately I didn't take it too seriously, why would I when the truth and facts regarding Ms Menopause are hidden from us by the medical world. I just kept working. December 2010 was my last period, the month of my fiftieth birthday. I always said that I didn't want to go into my fifties still dealing with periods, so I am thinking, "You beauty! All is on track."

In February 2011, the daughter had to move back home to have a major operation on a bone in her leg and the tendons in her foot. It put the girl out of action for more that six months. She had to endure what I call a "building site" on her leg that I nicknamed "Rambo". As horrible as it was, you really have to count your blessings. We saw quite a number of poor souls coming and going from the hospital with these bloody building sites that look like scaffolding attached to their heads! Scary. I was struggling with my skin, but not too badly, and had time off for my daughter's needs. Then I went back to work.

I was able to do six-hour shifts (thanks boss) so I was able to balance care for my daughter and earning some dollars. The daughter couldn't be on her own in the early stages, so we worked around her to ensure that someone was with her at all times. So on we went, caring for my daughter and working.

I noticed my face was starting to get a red glow to it and was starting to swell more and more. My work mates noticed too. When someone would mention the redness of my face, I used to just respond with, "Yeah, it's just my allergies." One morning in June 2011 I woke up and looked in a mirror. My face was twice its size, my eyes looked small and, honestly I was almost unrecognisable. I walked out and said to my brother, "Well I think it's time I went up to the hospital to get checked." Luckily he recognized my voice. At this time my daughter's girlfriend was staying. The daughter wouldn't be left alone, so off we went to the hospital.

As soon as the nurse saw me, I started crying. As she was testing my blood pressure, my arm was held straight out and up, and it was shaking like I had Parkinson's Disease. I was seen by a doctor and sent home on 25mg of steroids and a promise that he would get me to my allergist earlier than August. It didn't happen.

I was rostered on to work in other sections as they were short staffed. So this was the start of my life being taken over by Ms Menopause, the start of her affecting my life, my family, my earning power, my relationships, and my whole standing in life. On we went, caring for my daughter and me, living on antihistamines and steroids daily.

In August 2011 I went to see the allergist. I took my blood result readings with me. As he was looking at them he questioned what one was. I told him I was in menopause. He just said okay and pretty well acted as if it was neither here nor there.

At this time none of us, not my doctor, me, or the allergist had linked my exaggerated allergies to being a result of menopause. Well at least nobody told me they were linked. A normal allergy rate is 0 –

100, my rate was sitting at 13,000. High hey, but I wasn't too concerned as I thought the desensitization injections would deal with it. I was allergic to so much that when asked what I was allergic to I would just say, "Earth." It was easier than naming everything. I sat down one day and found if I took all the food that I was allergic to out of the equation, it would leave me only black cups of coffee. Knowing what I know now, and what you're going to discover about about the adrenal glands, I would have been left with a hot cup of water! My allergies are not just limited to food though. The allergies cover food including nuts, animals, chemicals, drugs, perfumes and just stuff. Aren't I the lucky one?

Funnily enough, I am still allergic to housework. They never seem to have found a cure for this one. Don't get me wrong, housework I do, but have always thought there are better things I could be doing with my time.

When I found out I was allergic to alcohol, well, imagine a little two year old throwing the biggest tantrum. Now imagine me. It's the first Friday night after a week of work that I haven't be able to yell, "Thank God it's Friday!" and put my brain in a box for a wee time while enjoy a few adult slurpies. There I was walking around the house cursing. "This is bullshit, I am a fifty-one year old woman. If I want to enjoy a few drinks now and then after a week at work I should bloody well be able too! Blah, blah, blah!" Yeah, not a pretty sight, but I have got use to it. Sort of. Well not really, but at the moment I have no choice. It's not just about the alcohol however, Ms Menopause has taken over every aspect of my life.

Now back to the allergist. My allergist explained that the desensitization needles that I had back in 1999 normally does a person through a life time, but 10% of the "allergy population" will need booster shots. I was one of them. Am I at all surprised? No. Of course I am one of the special 10% of the population! So off I went, from September 2011 until January 2012, to have five months of fortnightly booster shots. At least these needles are all natural things being injected into me. My daughter got through her traumatic experience and went back to her job and also started studying. Me? I was struggling.

I was still working, but was starting to have more time off. Not just a day or two, at times it was weeks. I was on a 6am start and would rock up with swollen eyes and face, not too bad, but enough to be noticed, waiting for the steroids and the antihistamines to kick in. Others and I started noticing blotches on my arm from the wrist to my elbow. These would bleed if bumped, so I started to bandage and put band-aids on my arms, partly to protect my skin, but mainly out of respect for my work mates. I keep my nails short. If I scratched this part of my arms it could cause the blotches.

It's a shame that I have to keep my nails short, I have always told my daughter that she comes from a long line of women with beautiful nails and the daughter has inherited this. Oh well, if that was all I had to whine about, I am doing marvellously well!

I say blotches but it's actually blood under the layer of skin. I did find out down the track that these red blotches were due to the long-term use of steroids. Apparently it causes thinning of the blood vessels. At their worst, if bumped they would bleed out. My face was red, my skin was dry and flaky. I had to moisturise more in one day than I had ever had to in my last fifty years, and sleep was becoming a very distant memory. As for the thinning of blood vessels, it couldn't be where no one could see it, could it? No! Nothing is ever subtle with me.

I look back now and am so thankful that the boss had asked me to cover for this section. It was away from the main building. I started at 6am and finished at 2pm, so I was able to just get in and out. I was also the only girl working with all men. They didn't care what I looked like. I could have turned up in my nana nightie with my socks and steel capped shoes on and crazy hair like Albert Einstein for all they cared. Okay, my hair always looks a bit crazy anyway. It was always great to see my girl mates in the main building though, I was struggling so much and it was becoming an effort to talk about it. Thank you all for asking and caring, but men, yeah they don't ask questions like women do. I miss my Thursday morning catch up with one of my girl mates, you know who you are, and miss chatting to some other work buddies as well.

I was also starting to lose money because of all the time I was having to take off. Oh and while I remember, rum balls sometimes have slivers of nut in them. I had a lovely little feast on them then had to have two days off work. It put me out of action for four days including my weekend. My energy levels fell. I was sitting on my lounge at home and felt so fatigued that I was falling asleep sitting up. I was later told by a nurse to always let someone know if this ever happens as my body could have been going into allergic shock. Strewth! I haven't touched a rum ball since.

I was also finding that I was so tired after finishing a shift that I had to concentrate on staying awake while driving home. I know that even without dealing with menopause, any one of us can be tired after a day's work, but this tiredness was different. I would start my shifts at 6am, 9am, 11am, 1pm, 3pm and 5pm. I was all over the place depending on which section I was working in. I wasn't new to this shift work, I had been doing it and enjoying it for a while up to this point. The tiredness I was feeling was consuming, I really felt I needed to stop the car to let myself have a snooze on the way home, which was only fifteen to twenty minutes away depending on traffic.

Because of this "to the core" tiredness, I really was not compassionate towards others at times. I stopped off at our corner shop on the way home and a child of about three years old was chucking a tantrum. The shopkeeper said to me, "Oh poor sweetheart, she is tired." I looked at this three year old and all I could respond with was, "Yeah, and she isn't the only one! I wish I could chuck myself down on the floor sobbing because I am exhausted and have someone pick me up, take me home and put me to bed!"

So there you go, competing with a three year old as to who is more tired and who is more worthy of being carried lovingly back to the car! She won of course. Old enough to know how to get her own way, not old enough to drive. Yeah, I see what you are doing missy! Suck it up for all it's worth now sweetie 'cause in approx forty-seven years time, not many people are going to give a crap about how bloody tired you are! Try that act then and you will be left on that floor as they are turning the lights off and locking up the shop. Even better you may be escorted off the premises by some people in uniform who have brought you a not so fashionable white jacket with really long arms that can be wrapped around to the back of you, to wear. Yeah, I'd like to see that! And that ladies, was a prime example of a woman not supporting a future woman. Hopefully though in forty-seven years time, this little three year old's journey with Ms Menopause will be a lot easier.

I also had more blood tests after the completion of the five months of fortnightly booster allergy shots in January 2012 to see where my allergy rate was sitting. It had gone up from 13,000 to 16,000. Hmm, okay, I'm confused.

I also knew within myself that all I was dealing with had only started since Ms Menopause arrived. She was at the top of my hit list, but not one person I had dealt with in the medical world up to this point had told me that. The only thing that I had been told is that I am forty-three something-or-other in menopause, so I held onto that.

My dealings with different medical people and different departments may have been easier if I had thrown Ms Menopause down to the bottom of the list, but had I swept Ms Menopause under the rug like that, I would have let myself, my daughter and all women down.

I kept soldering on as best as I could, still living on steroids and anti-histamines and having days off work, but in June 2012 I had to have a week off. I was struggling at home then on the 30th of June I went to bed but I could not get comfortable. It felt like someone had their knuckles pressing in my lower back. It was extremely uncomfortable and it hurt. I was scared. I thought maybe there was a problem with my kidneys. I also started to crave salt. So back up to the hospital. This time I was admitted. My steroids were "upped" to 50mg, I was given a drug that felt FAB-U-LOUS! I had an intravenous line in each hand, I was red, swollen, sobbing and my skin was hurting. Gorgeous eh! My daughter said that when she visited me, my head was three times its normal size. I would start a conversation then forget mid-sentence what I was saying and just start crying. So horrible. I had people who wanted to come and visit me but I had to say no, I was just not up to seeing anyone outside of my immediate family. The daughter would say at times when she was younger, "Hostipal isn't much fun, is it mum?" No it isn't daughter.

I told the doctor about the knuckling feeling and that I was craving salt. I asked if she could check my kidneys, but all blood tests came back showing my kidneys were good. Okay. The doctor originally wanted me to stay one more night for observation but I just wanted to get home. This was the first and only time, apart from the birth of my daughter twenty-one years ago, that I had been admitted to hospital, even with the childhood asthma.

The medication I had been given when I had been admitted in June 2012 was doing it's job, I was out of there, I needed to escape, yes, escape from the sweet old nurse who was taking care of me. I say sweet because she was. I gave her the nickname "Clarence" after the old angel in training in the movie, "It's a Wonderful Life". But after the umpteenth time of trying to take blood out of my hand at the doctor's request, I had to put a stop to it. I have what I call "good man hands", good healthy veins for the taking, but this sweet old nurse just couldn't seem to jab one correctly. After being a patient - patient, get it - for a while and enduring the pain, I had to put a stop to it saying, "Enough, no more!"

I must have thundered this out like bloody Thor as all eyes turned to me. Even my visitors' eyes widened, looking shocked and scared.

The doctor finally came and took the required blood in one attempt. I asked why they needed another lot of blood. The doctor explained that the first lot of blood results came back looking pretty scary, and they just needed to check it all again as sometimes when they take blood, something can happen and give false results. Okay! I now understood why an intravenous line was put in both hands, and I walked out of there with a souvenir of my visit, a bloody gigantic bruise on my left hand.

It's a Wonderful Life—This movie was made in 1946, with the great Jimmy Stewart. It's about a man who, due to the unfortunate turn of events in his life, contemplates suicide. An old bumbling angel in training is sent to show him the world and how it would be if he had never been born. I try and watch it at Christmas time each year. It is a lovely movie that reminds us we are all meant to be here, and that there is a ripple effect we all have on each other, and it doesn't matter how bad things seem at times, they are never bad enough to end your life. Clarence the angel does his job well. Jimmy Stewart, in the movie, sees clarity and realizes that what is really important in life is loved ones. And Clarence earns his wings.

I ended up having another two weeks off work. It was hard. Just having a shower hurt my skin, and the process of moisturizing was exhausting. I would shuffle from the shower to the lounge, sit down, and then wait for someone to feed me. I was hardly sleeping, and when I did it was at all the wrong times.

There were times through all this that I actually thought I might die. It sounds dramatic I know, but I did think it. I even gave my family the "death talk" and asked them to keep on loving each other and keep being there for each other, blah blah blah. I was also craving the sun. We would sit out in the backyard catching some rays. Once, while sitting out there with my best mate, I said, "This is like the scene out of *Beaches*, the one when the two best mates are sitting looking out to the ocean," well we were looking at my back fence, "before the sick one dies." That didn't go down too well. I found out I was also deficient in Vitamin D, hence the craving for the sun.

I went back to work the following week, the 9th of July 2012, I couldn't afford not to. I was feeling better. Sitting on 50mg of steroids gives you a pretty good dose of energy and makes your skin look gorgeous and plump, even though you know it's not doing you any good long term. I remember praying for more time off. Long term, I knew the steroids and all the rest were just a band-aid. I knew I was going to crash and burn again. I needed more time to heal and take care of myself and work out what was actually happening to me.

Because of circumstances within the business, I applied for voluntary redundancy due to my genuine health issues. I walked away from the job on the 17th of July with a package that was a godsend, and the finances are still looking after themselves, for now. I just have to look after myself. As I have always said, "Never underestimate the power of prayer." I was quite sad to walk from my job, I didn't want to leave but I had no choice.

Talking about finances, as much as I was very fortunate to end my job with this money in my pocket, as time goes on, I am accessing all sorts of funds that should not have to be used at this age. I have also had to use savings that I was planning to use for my "bucket list". The ripple effect is huge. I do know, and am very thankful, that I am still very fortunate compared to others. Our family home is secure and I own the car. It may not be the latest model, but I love it. The car will always stay. I will keep putting money into it, as it belonged to my sister.

I have family support emotionally and at times financially, when waiting on the next lot of funds to be released. I have, like many others, moments I need to borrow from Peter to pay Paul. To the young ones who are reading this, that means to put off paying one bill to pay another. So yeah, Ms Menopause cannot only affect your health, she can grab a hold of your whole life and toss you in the gutter. I just thank God that I have loved ones supporting me, for without it, my life at this point could have been so horribly different. Again, it sounds very dramatic, but for some women this could be the reality of their lives given the constant battering Ms Menopause can inflict. It just saddens me deeply to think there are women out there who may be doing this on their own.

I also know for a fact that there are women who are dragging the chain in the workplace purely due to Ms Menopause. I know women who are struggling to keep their much wanted and needed jobs because Ms Menopause is starting to engulf them. With correct information a lot earlier, this need not happen.

Chapter 7

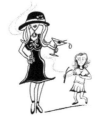

CENTRELINK…OH DEAR!

What happens to those women who haven't got support, or who can't afford to pay their bills, if Ms Menopause brings them to their knees? I know we have Centrelink here in Australia, but not once have I seen anything that caters for any woman who is dealing with menopause. I have also found that when you are really sick there is no way you have the health or energy to try and jump through hoops. Even when you are not sick, those who really need the support don't get it at times while those who know how to rort the system get it all.

When another very wise and gorgeous mate of mine, you know who you are, knew I'd left my job because of illness, she insisted that I register with Centrelink, if for nothing else just to get the healthcare card, and yes I am finding out that medications and treatments can be expensive. I did go in and give them the doctor's reports. First, they didn't put me on a disability payment, no, I was put on a Newstart payment. This payment is for those looking for work. Why? Why was I not put on a Disability Payment? I say Disability Payment because as far as I know, there is not a Menopause Payment and I think that needs to change!

Did they think I was pretending to be sick? Was I not taken seriously because the word "Menopause" was mentioned? Or is it because they had no category to slot me into? I don't know. Because of the payment I received from having to leave my work, I was given a payment of $70 a fortnight. Fair enough I say, I actually wasn't even expecting that. I don't want their money if I can support myself.

Secondly, because I was on a Newstart payment, I had to get three monthly certificates from my doctor to say I was still unable to work. The latest of these covered up to mid-December 2012. I was receiving letters from an employment agency in October 2012 advising me I had to attend an appointment. I didn't go. I also received another notification stating I had to report all of my earnings in November 2012. I sent them a short email asking why, when the certificate I submitted to them from my doctor covered up to the middle of December 2012. I didn't get a call back as requested, but a couple of weeks later I got a letter from them saying I didn't have to report until Feb 2013. Ok, I thought, finally sense has arrived.

A week later I received a letter informing me that my payment had been stopped because I had not attended an appointment with that damn employment agency. I don't really recall which one. To finish this saga, I then received another letter from the employment agency saying that if I did not attend an appointment in January 2013, my payment would be stopped. Oh okay, so you are going to stop it? Too late matey, someone got in before you.

Wow, it's not finished yet, can you believe it? This is moving into the New Year but I want to keep this joyful saga together. So the $70 a fortnight Centrelink originally gave me was stopped mid-December 2012. I received a call, well they left a message. It was the employment agency girl again, later in January 2013. She said she wasn't too sure what was happening about me and was confused. She advised me that my payment had been stopped but I was still attached to their records. She requested that I ring her back so I could sort it all. I didn't ring her back.

For a split second I thought I will make that call and straighten her out, but then I thought, stuff it! It's not my job to sort this crap out. They are the employment agency, they should have a direct link with each other. You two services get paid to brain storm this, so sort it out. I don't give a rat's backside how confused you are in relation to me, stand in line because you wouldn't be the first, but it's not my job to sort your job. This just adds unnecessary stress. This sort of crap is bad enough when you are well, but when you are sick, it's not acceptable. Even when I was caring for my sister and dad, the Carer's Allowance was offered to me but I didn't accept it, have you seen the paperwork involved in getting this payment? Back then it was the size of a novel, so I didn't bother, I wasn't going to put my time and energy into that when it was time and energy needed and wanted for my family members. It is an insult to all those who want to get on with giving quality and quantity care time to their loved ones in their final stages of their lives.

I know this system needs to be protected, but it seems to me that our Centrelink system doesn't really look after it's own too well. You, Centrelink, also have to have compassion for those who are sick, caring for the sick, or are just having a tough time in their lives. Centrelink and I have gone our separate ways. I haven't got the energy or health to have to deal with all that again. I now just have to get this employment agency out of my life.

While I am on the subject, our government needs to find a way of incorporating menopause leave into the work place. The Medical World, Centrelink and our government have not considered women dealing with menopause at all. Why not?

Big News! Guess what? I have gone my separate way from Centrelink, but they have not finished with me yet. I received notice saying that if I didn't report my earnings from November 2012 to February 2013, they were going to take back payments that I had received from November 2012, even though my doctor's certificate covered up until December 2012.

You have to be joking! It is so ridiculous, it's laughable, it's nearly worth going to jail for, good luck guys getting the November 2012 payment of $70.42 back, even though I was covered up to mid-December. We all know what happens when we say, "It's the principle of the matter." I don't mind giving them money back if needed, but I'm sure not going to give my money just for the hell of it. Geez almighty!

So no doubt I will end up in jail and all because bloody Ms Menopause came a-knocking. Exciting. Oh and a message to that very wise and gorgeous mate of mine who demanded I go to Centrelink to get the card to help with expenses, I expect you to be my first visitor if I land in jail!

N.B. I am seeing a happy ending may be in sight for this Centrelink saga so a big thank you to those two women who work for Centrelink who have taken this on for me and are sorting it out.

I have now been off work for five months. I know now that I am dealing with menopause and all of the symptoms, as well as the exacerbation of allergies, so another phase starts. But at least I don't have to worry about work, or about money too much, well not yet. I am fighting to get healthy, happy and old and to get *me* back!

But first I want to say I am not attempting to hold onto my youth. If I wanted to look twenty at eighty years of age, that would be nobody's business, but I am not done and dusted at fifty-one and I refuse to accept the fact that women in their fifties have to feel at times like, "Well that's that, it's gone to crap now, just accept the fact that you are old." The thing is though, I am not old, I am older. I should not be shuffling around like a 100 year old because of menopause.

I walked into this next phase of my life with no knowledge of what was coming. I walked in with a gigantic bag full of pure ignorance.

Chapter 8

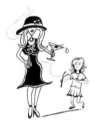

HRT, OH GOODY! NOT!

Before being admitted to hospital, I had been on a herbal tablet for menopause. When my doctor told me in 2010 that I was heading into menopause before my period stopped, this is how the conversation went:

Me: Oh am I?

Doc: Yes.

Me: Ok.

That was it. We then had a quick chat about the roller coaster effect. I can't remember when I spoke to him about the herbal stuff for menopause, but I remember being adamant I wasn't going to touch HRT. I had heard too many horror stories about it and some very sad stories too. I saw him in the week following my stay in hospital and he suggested HRT. I wasn't happy about it but it seemed to be my only option. Meanwhile the allergies were still not being linked to Ms Menopause. And so it was arranged.

I came home with my box of gel sachets, read the pamphlet and started. I had to rub a gel sachet into my thigh, I just had to alternate thighs daily. After a week I was already getting confused. Which bloody thigh is it today? I thought I would look into this HRT a bit more.

I read that women who had had a hysterectomy only needed the gel. Women who still had all their girly bits intact were to add ten days of progesterone into the mix. When a woman who still has all her reproductive organs uses the gel only, it can thicken the lining of the womb and cause endometrial cancer. What the…? My womb was still intact! Back to the doctor and home again with the progesterone tablets in hand. Now what did he say? Ten days of gel and the rest progesterone, or gel daily and ten days of the other and which bloody thigh am I up to?

I did do it properly but it was so confusing at times. It didn't take long before I started bleeding, or should I say haemorrhaging. It sure felt like that to me, type AB+ please! I didn't know that was going to happen. I obviously didn't read the information properly and I do remember reading something about spotting, so after eighteen months of no period, the HRT gave me a period again. Not just a period either, it was the mother of all periods. Just how much blood do we have in our bodies?

I was on HRT for three months and not only did I bleed pretty well constantly for a while, I was also bloated. I still am but the bloating on HRT was horrible. I felt nauseated, the headaches were horrible and I was even more tired. When the bleeding didn't stop, my doctor said to cease the HRT. Yes please, I don't know who was more scared or bloody terrified, my doctor or me!

After a while the bleeding stopped. I know now there are other forms of HRT that can be taken, but I will never, ever go near it again. Thank God no damage was done. I hope. After getting over the shock of it all, of course I had to do some further investigating. This is what I found:

HRT used to be called ERT (Oestrogen Replacement Therapy). In 1975 The New England Journal of Medicine studied endometrial cancer. Women taking ERT for under seven years were five times more at risk of getting endometrial cancer. Over seven years usage of ERT, a woman's chance of getting endometrial cancer shot up to fourteen times higher. I also read they were debating as to whether endometrial cancer is a man made cancer caused by ERT. Interesting but bloody scary. I don't know what the outcome of that was.

They added synthetic progesterone to ERT and its new name is HRT. Huh? I need to ask my doctor a question. I thought HRT had no progesterone in it and that was why I had to add in ten days of it. I will get back to you on that one in my "I'm Confused" chapter.

The American Cancer Society, after a thirteen-year study, found women who had been on HRT under eleven years, had a 40% higher ovarian cancer risk. For women who had been on HRT over eleven years, their risk of ovarian cancer rose to 70%. HRT side effects include: breast cancer, depression, strokes, lupus and heart attacks to mention a few. I do understand that with a woman's most desperate and debilitating suffering at the hands of Ms Menopause, HRT may be seen as their only choice regardless of the side affects. Look at me, I was given it as my only option and I did that to my body for three months even though I had been so against it.

Come on Medical World. There has to be a better way. Women today are still being used as guinea pigs when it comes to their health. My daughter and women the world over have the right to know the facts. It is their body, and their right. They say women are living longer due to HRT, yeah but again at what cost to their health?

My doctor organised another appointment with my allergist. This time, armed with some knowledge, I also put myself on their cancellation list! My blood test showed my allergy rate was now sitting at 22,250. Yeah, getting scary now, no wonder I ended up in hospital. I went and saw my allergist again in August 2012. He did the normal allergy testing, and since August I have to have monthly desensitization injections for a year, until July 2013. You know, you put your faith in the medical world and expect them to do the best for you. I again asked this first allergist - notice the "first?"- whether he thought that the reason my allergies keep rising was due to menopause. I gave him the chance, but once again it was dismissed.

Why did I stay with that allergist? Well like I said, I thought we put our faith in them and they will look after us. We will see how we travel, health wise, through this year of injections. For now though I will give you my inexpert opinion. I am not as special as I thought, I am not a part of that 10% club that needs booster shots. The exacerbation of my allergies is purely and simply because Ms Menopause arrived on my doorstep.

The allergist though, for the first time since I had dealt with him all the way back in 1999, took blood tests. I didn't think much about it, when you are not well sometimes you just don't ask why. It had taken all my strength just to keep the appointment. My doctor later told me the allergist was testing for "lupus" which came back negative. It would be interesting though to see what percentage of that 10% club are women and what age group they fall into.

Chapter 9

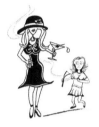

DRUGS, DRUGS & MORE BLOODY DRUGS

Before Ms Menopause knocked, the only drugs I ever willingly put in my body throughout my lifetime were The Pill - I used to gag every time I put it in my mouth, I certainly don't miss that drug, - and alcohol. I certainly do miss that drug. Oh I also had a puff of a joint when I was eighteen, but never touched it again. I didn't enjoy it and didn't like the feel of it, so I just stayed with my good mates Scotch and Chardy and my holiday mates Cocktails.

The last drug I have willingly put in my body is ciggies. I have been a smoker, a non smoker, a social smoker, cut down to a few-a-day smoker, a closet smoker, hey, I even gave it up for three months because I got bored with it and had no desire to smoke throughout my pregnancy. I have done hypnotherapy, acupuncture, the chewing gum, patches, cold turkey, blah blah blah. I am not writing about this to say yay or nay in regard to smoking. But if you haven't started, why bother!

I did however, in fairness, want to have a look into this habit of mine. This is what I found in relation to menopause: Smoking can put a woman into earlier menopause. Now I was fifty-one after twelve months of no periods. Apparently, this is the average age for women, so yeahnah. Smoking is supposedly giving women harsher and more frequent hot flushes. Hot flushes, for me, are not a big one. I once felt flushed at the checkout, and my eyes started to fill up with tears. I also, on another day, suddenly felt overwhelmed and I, as my daughter put it, "lost it." I cried in the fruit and vege aisle, but I didn't get a flushed face, nothing is subtle with me.

I have also met a handful of women who say that they "sailed" through menopause. After congratulating them and being genuinely happy for them I had to ask, "Do you smoke?" Some did, some didn't. So that sort of threw my own little "in fairness" investigation out the window. Even I, as a layperson, realize that only asking a handful of women is not a "you beaut" scientifically proven study, so I will continue to ask that question. I actually don't smoke much anymore anyway, I can't bloody afford them! Too busy spending my money on medications and on specialist appointments who don't bulk bill! Thank you to those who did at times bulk bill and a gigantic thank you to my doctor. It has been appreciated. Even though you are not an expert on menopause, you are a wonderful doctor and at times you have taken the stress out of having to find the funds to see you.

I do know that smoking depletes your body of vitamin C and I do know that at fifty-one if I want a ciggie now and then, I am bloody well going to have it. To be honest I look forward to the day when I can once again enjoy a scotch with it, because that day will come. Won't it?

I also think it is insulting to all those women who have never smoked but are still experiencing debilitating flushes. How does the Medical Community explain that? Well it can't. So stop trying to always blame a woman's struggle throughout menopause on other things Medical Community. It's insulting, annoying and not acceptable anymore!

These are the drugs, up to now, I have had to use since Ms Menopause's arrival. I put them on me, in me and carry them with me:

Three types of steroid creams, for face, body and the big guns for when my skin gets out of hand, applied daily or twice a day.

- Prednisone (steroid): since June 2011, I have had to take 50mg, 25mg, 10mg, 5mg, back up to 25mg etc, taken daily.
- Zantac Tablets: I have to take this to counteract the effect of the Prednisone, taken daily.
- Paraffin Ointment: moisturises my skin after I put the steroid creams on, after each shower daily, more on a daily basis depending on how my skin is.
- Sandrena: The HRT gel I was on for three months. We all know how much fun that was.
- Provera: This is the progesterone I had to mix in with the Sandrena. Never, Ever, Again!
- Antihistamines: all types and strengths daily. In the early days of using these I had a reaction to one type, go figure. Make sure you read what is in these before you use them, you may have an allergy to one of the ingredients. If it wasn't so serious it would be laughable. What? I have to take another antihistamine to settle down the effect of the antihistamine I just took?
- Endep: These are sleeping tablets. I chose not to continue taking them, they zonk me out, I don't want them to become my normal.
- Desensitization needles: Five months of fortnightly vaccinations from September 2011 to January 2012, and for now the year of monthly vaccinations from August 2012 to July 2013.
- Antibiotics: For the earaches and infections.
- Ear drops: Two types, as I had a reaction to the first type. Yeah no joke, it's getting embarrassing just admitting to it.
- Ear Cream: My earaches and swelling of ears continue, yes you get the full story a bit later.

I spoke to my doctor and told him I didn't want to depend on antibiotics all the time, so we are trying a cream ointment that I just put in my ears three times a day. "The one that hasn't got penicillin in it please," because as we know, I am allergic to it. We will see how this ointment works out.

I became a Panadol user for the HRT headaches, for those menopause headaches, for the earache and swelling-of-my-ears-headaches. Geez, I feel I need to pop a few Panadol now. Just thinking about it all gives me a headache.

With all the medications and creams I need on a daily basis, I need to be of sound mind to keep up with it all.

My doctor also spoke to me regarding anti-depressant tablets, but he didn't even get to write the script out for this one. Again, I don't want it to become my normal.

Chapter 10

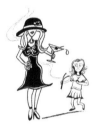

MY LITTLE BLACK BOOK
DEPRESSION & SUICIDE

All that I have had to deal with since Ms Menopause knocked has been a challenge and at times scary, but nothing has scared me more than depression.

This little black book is a record of my struggle with depression. I started writing in this book when I knew something was not right with my thoughts, but I had no idea how big and scary my thoughts would become. I get angry and worried when it is said by a so-called expert that menopause does not cause menopause-induced depression as such, or when it is not taken seriously by the medical community. Angry because menopause-induced depression is a very real thing, and worried because woman are again made to feel that what they are going through is not real, and they are not believed.

I find it gobsmacking that some of the experts have such a flippant attitude towards it.

It is a fact that the two hormones oestrogen and progesterone are produced in much lower amounts during menopause which does affect the serotonin levels in a woman's brain which leads to depression.

Many women are committing suicide or attempting suicide in this phase of their lives. Until now, I had never encountered depression. I have been sad, upset, cried and grieved, but depression was something I never understood, or to be quite honest, it was something I didn't have to understand. I did support a young friend once who was dealing with it, so I did research it, but I was still on the outside of it. I know my daughter has supported a few friends through it.

Now suicide, well this makes me cry at times. Suicide does that to me, it upsets me that a human being decides to end their life. I have personally only known one person who has committed suicide. I was in my twenties and he was a work buddy. My daughter though, has lost and almost lost friends to suicide.

I always thought suicide was sad and selfish. Sad because the person had no one to talk to and they felt this was their only option, selfish because of loved ones left behind with the "whys" and "what ifs" that they carry with them for the rest of their life.

The following are my writings in my little black book. They are very personal and at times very raw, hopefully though any woman reading this will feel better knowing "it's not just you" and that what you are going through is very, very real, regardless of what you may be told by the experts:

- I am scared sometimes that my family will get fed up with me. I am becoming a burden to them. I am having thoughts that my family may be better off without me.
- I am nothing but a burden. I am nobody. I have nothing. I wish my mum was here to talk to.

- I think I am heading into depression. I never knew depression could creep up and grab you and you would sink into it. I am dissolving and disappearing. I am scared! I have to fight it.
- It's scary! Oh my God! I have always been a strong person, but the depression just crept up on me. Depression is not me! I never knew depression had a mind of its own.
- I am tired. I just want to wake up healthy and be me again. I can't continue to live like this.
- Oh my God I have been thinking about suicide! I am scared that the depression will be stronger than me. I have to fight it. I have to be stronger than it.
- I just realised how easy it could be to commit suicide when depressed, it's like another me in my head telling me to just do it and that I am useless. That is depression doing that, not me!
- It is such a lonely place to be.
- Dear God, please don't let me go crazy and please don't let me commit suicide. I want to live and be healthy. I want to be here for me. I want to be here for my family. Please help me to get back to the strong woman, mum, sister, friend and person I used to be. Please help me to find me again. Amen.

Pretty dramatic, but this is how it was for me, I understand now how one can become nothing when in this state. The depression and thoughts of suicide are very strong and scary and very, very, real. I had never known that depression could have a mind of its own. Sounds strange? I will explain. My doctor prescribed sleeping tablets, and as I said before, I am not taking them. One day, out of nowhere, the thought, "Just take a handful of those tablets, your family will be better off without you," just rang in my head. I then thought, no way. If depression makes me take those tablets, I will be ringing triple zero as soon as I swallow them! Bizarre and terrifying.

I had other thoughts, but the main thing I was starting to notice was that my worst thoughts were when I was alone. It was when the family wasn't home, or when I was alone waiting to see my doctor, or when I was in the next aisle away from my daughter at the shops or if I was driving alone or when a mate had just left after coming over for a coffee. What I also discovered was that depression is a coward, not brave enough to show its ugly head when I was surrounded by loved ones and others.

I sat at home one night thinking, "Is it just me?" So off I went to research it. I was shocked to see menopause is a peak time for women to attempt or actually suicide. I went and grabbed my little black book then wrote in it "FEK...OFF depression! I am not going to kill myself just because YOU want me to!"

I only spoke to my close loved ones when I did understand it and realized I was dealing with menopause-induced depression. I have written that depression is a symptom of menopause, but I would never have imagined the depth of despair and the thoughts of suicide are so, so scary until I dealt with it myself. I still deal with it, but now that I understand it I am mostly in charge of it. I have days even now when it rears up again and I struggle through with it, but it is not stronger than me anymore, well at the moment. Again, never underestimate the power of prayer.

It's scary too, that at its worst I didn't talk about it. I did say to a mate in the early stages, I think I am heading into depression, but that was it. At this stage we had a quick chat, but I didn't know it was heading in a direction that would become terrifying. How did I know I was heading into depression when I really did not know much about it? I don't know, I think it was all the thoughts that started off as subtle, quick, soft thoughts about being a burden, then they became louder, more frequent and more controlling.

At the peak of this depression, I had booked an appointment with my doctor for my pap-smear test. As I walked in and sat down, I just started sobbing. In amongst the sobbing I was saying, "I am so sorry, this is not me." My doctor then asked me had I been having any suicidal thoughts, which surprised me. All I could say was, "Yeah, but I wouldn't do anything." As I said this, I wasn't convinced I wouldn't do anything.

My doctor wanted to prescribe anti-depressants but I didn't get a script. My doctor understands my decision. He also now monitors my mental state. As one would imagine, the pap-smear test was rescheduled, but at least I scored some jellybeans from my doctor's lolly jar!

I have never had to depend on medication for depression at any time throughout my life and I really don't want it to become my "normal" now, but I do understand that medication can save lives, and bring quality and happiness back into peoples' lives.

There are different types of depression. I didn't even know that! In regard to my personal dealings with my menopause-induced depression this is what I have learnt:

Depression can creep up on you in a horrible, subtle way until it's in your thoughts every day, taking over. Depression has a strength and mind of its own. Depression makes you feel you are nothing, and depression isolates you.

During my journey with depression, I wondered whether it is the person who willingly commits suicide or whether it is the depression taking over? Sounds really strange, but as said earlier, if I had popped those sleeping tablets and then rung triple zero after, I would have been admitted to hospital, I think, for attempted suicide. Many people think, "Oh they did it for attention." Well, I can think of better ways to get attention, there would have been no attention seeking on my part, I want to live! It simply would have been the fact that the depression was stronger than me.

As I mentioned, throughout it I was not talking about it. I have heard that when people commit suicide, they don't talk about it, they just do it. During the greatest part of my battle and the suicidal thoughts, I didn't talk to anyone either, I just kept writing it all down in my little black book. Why didn't I talk to anyone? Why didn't I scream out to my family, "HELP ME, I AM THINKING OF SUICIDE!"

Not talking about it wasn't a deliberate thing. I wasn't consciously hiding it, I wasn't ashamed of it, I didn't even fully understand it. In a way it becomes your normal, even when you know it's not normal. It was only when I realised that it wasn't just me that I started to control it. Also know this, knowledge is power. This depression will put your mind in another place and it isolates you. It isolates you physically - I sleep more at times and am anti-social; emotionally - it strips you of your confidence and self worth; mentally - I felt like I was going crazy and was scared I was going to be weaker than it; and it also isolated my mind - it changes your thought patterns.

I did have people to talk to, I just didn't. I didn't keep it a secret, I just didn't tell anyone. I was so consumed by it, but honestly never really thought to speak out loud about it. Loved ones are cluey though. My brother said that he thought I might be depressed, and then straight away asked when my next appointment with my doctor was. My daughter would just come and give me a kiss or a hug for no reason, but it was always at a time when it was needed. I would receive an sms from my mate saying she was on her way over with coffee, just out of the blue, at the right time.

I have a mate who I don't see much but we email. She would send an, "Are you okay?" email if she hadn't heard any news from me for a day or two. Now this friend doesn't know about my battle with depression, but her emails always came at the right time. Keep them all coming my friend, when I check my inbox I always look forward to reading them, and thank you for your wonderful friendship.

I truly didn't think my loved ones could see it. Even though I am dealing with menopause symptoms, along with the exacerbation of my allergies, they saw that something was taking me away.

When I did a bit of research on this, I read of a grandmother who had committed suicide and I'm sure there are many more. I am also sure there are many cases of women who have attempted suicide, where the reasons have just been put down to their mental state, with no thought that Ms Menopause is behind it.

Another wife and mum had changed since the onset of menopause two years prior. Before menopause she had been a bubbly, lively, gentle woman and had been happy. This woman was now fifty-two years old. Her doctor had prescribed antidepressants, but she would not take them for a week at a time as she did not like drugs. She was also afraid to take HRT because she had high blood pressure. Menopause caused her to have severe mood swings. Mostly she would stare at the TV. When her husband was talking she would hear him without listening.

The couple had just returned from a trip and the wife seemed happy enough. One morning the husband had left for work. He had thought his wife was fine and she had even asked him what he wanted for dinner. The wife had previously said, "I wish I could disappear in a puff of smoke." Well she did. She loaded the cartridge into a shotgun and placed it to the side of her head. The husband discovered his beautiful wife's body when he came home from work. After losing his wife this man said, "I wish more people realized the damaging effects that menopause can have on women."

The inquest was told that the woman had been very good at hiding her depression and her GP didn't believe her to be suicidal. Recording a suicide verdict the coroner said, "It is quite clear that was not a cry for help. I am convinced [she] was aware of the immediate consequences of her actions and that she took those actions voluntarily while depressed."

I believe this woman was dealing with the same menopause-induced depression that I have been struggling with, so this is what I say: Do you think for a moment this woman wanted to pull that trigger? No, she didn't. Do you think for a moment this woman wanted to leave her life, her wonderful husband and her two gorgeous children? No, she didn't. I believe the depression was stronger than her.

The coroner said this woman took these actions voluntarily while depressed. No she didn't. This woman didn't do this voluntarily. The word voluntarily means it was a choice. No one ever suicides voluntarily with depression, rather, depression kidnaps your mind and takes over.

The inquest was also told this woman was very good at hiding her depression. I have learnt it is not a deliberate "hiding" of depression. This woman was scared and fighting for her life. I found it interesting that her GP did not think she was suicidal, but someone prescribed the anti-depressants and you can't just stop and start taking them. I assume the doctor didn't know she was doing this, and if he did he should have been concerned. The medical world needs to get off its backside and stop trivializing and being so flippant about menopause.

Chapter 11

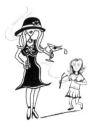

AND OTHER THINGS

My mate had just moved over to Stradbroke Island and thought it would be good for me to head over with her at times. I did go over for a couple of days, but never went back again in the six months she was there. The whole thought of it was exhausting. The time I did go over, I had to carry all my medications with me, everything becomes an effort.

I had also booked a weeks holiday at beautiful Tangalooma resort on Moreton Island. I have been taking my daughter there since she was five. We have not gone over for a few years but it's my favourite holiday spot. The day arrived to head over but I was too unwell to go. On the fourth day of the booking my daughter and my mate came to me and said that we were heading over for the remaining days as they thought it would be good for me. It was really push and shove for me, but I did go over with my best mate to finish the two days we had left of the booking.

When I first got off the launch I felt for a second like the old me. It was lovely to be back, we had fun and a few scotches that I knew I would suffer for later, and we did a lot of chatting, but we only stayed one night, as I wasn't well and really needed to be at home.

Ms Menopause has stripped me of many little things that we all take for granted. I do not know how I am going to feel until I wake up in the morning or whenever I have been able to catch some sleep. Getting out of bed can be a mammoth task, waking up swollen and groggy and getting ready to have a shower takes a huge psychological effort, as my energy is low and I know as soon as the water hits my skin it will hurt. It is difficult to eat when not hungry, but I have to as I have medication to take and I have to eat just to survive. Putting the creams on my body, then moisturising is exhausting. I don't do much cooking anymore, my brother does - you are a chef bro! - and my daughter will cook a meal at times.

Just doing the washing up can take me forever as I need to sit down constantly. I used to shop for groceries online, but now that I am off work I thought it would be good to actually go to the shops. But I can't do the shopping on my own and I can't carry heavy items so the daughter comes with me or does the shopping for me. Occasionally I have done a small grocery shop, but at times I have become overwhelmed and just wanted to run out of there.

I have cancelled social events and my social life is pretty well "nada". Some days when I have a bit of energy and my skin isn't too swollen, red or flaky, I go and have coffee with a mate, but it has to be close to home. It doesn't happen often and has become more of a non-event as time goes on. I used to love the build up to Christmas, work would get busier and I always loved getting out into the shops finalising presents. This year I did it all online.

As for the depression, it is still quite surreal and very scary looking back at it's peak to remember I was contemplating writing goodbye letters to my loved ones. I am still at a stage with it where I wouldn't turn my back on it. I am very aware that it could pop up out of nowhere.

The one thing I still do well is drive, but if I drive too much, it tires me out. Before Ms Menopause came along I would have considered this amount of driving to be only a little bit. Sometimes I get jittery and don't drive for days. Some mornings I am jittery and fidgety from the moment I awake. I am guessing the nervous tension symptom is to blame for this. At times, family have kindly driven me to appointments and places I need to be. I can't deal with stress at the moment. I know I am not the mum, sister or best friend I used to be. I am not the friend I used to be to my other mates. I am quite anti-social, not because I want to be, I just haven't got the energy or health to be the mate I once was, and I just don't have the energy or health to be there physically or emotionally for anyone.

I have gone from being a woman who worked hard, had a good social life, loved laughing out loud, and slept pretty damn well, to a woman who had to walk away from her job, who has a non- existent social life, who has fewer big roars of laughter anymore—and sleep, well, depending on what day it is, what is that?

Oh, and let's talk about crying. I have never been a big crier, although I had always believed that a good cry is good for you, but geez! I sobbed in front of my doctor, I have cried in the fruit and vege aisle, I cry sometimes because this journey of ill health just gets too big for me, I have cried because I miss me at times, I have cried because the physical pain just hurts, I have cried as I know how it is affecting my family and some days I just cry.

Now in saying all this, I know I am still fortunate and I count my blessings every day. I wake up. I did not take my own life and leave my family and friends behind. I may be feeling like I am breathing yet am not alive, but I am still here. I get tired of the constant fight with it at times but I know someone out there is doing it a lot worse than me. I am loved and those closest have shown me that I am worthy of being cared for and looked after. Thank you loved ones, without all your support and love this journey would have been a hell of a lot harder.

You are the reason I am still here, why would I want to leave the best family in the whole entire universe?

Time to march onward to the next obstacles Ms Menopause threw at me. "What there is more?" I hear you say. Oh yes, indeedy!

Earaches: In mid October 2012 I was starting to get twinges of pain in my ears, just short quick stabs of pain. My ears were sore to touch and I could feel and hear that my left ear was blocking and swelling up and the pain was becoming constant. The left side of my face also was swollen just in the ear region in my cheek, so as you can imagine, a very attractive look! The right ear was a bit sore but nothing compared to the left ear. I went off to my doctor and returned home with eardrops. As I started using them, I noticed I was starting to get welts on my face. I was having a reaction to them! I stopped the drops, the ear settled down and I just waited for the welts to go.

About a week later, my right ear started blocking up and the pain was hideous. I walked out into the lounge room and just cried. You have to be joking! What doesn't kill you is supposed to make you stronger, but geez almighty, enough is enough! I had to laugh though, when I was crying in the lounge room, the daughter came over and gave me a hug and said, "We still love you mum, even if you look like Dumbo." Thank you daughter, I think, for making me giggle.

Back to the doctor. I came home with new and improved eardrops and antibiotics. They did the job, but this went on for a month. To be honest, as I am typing right now, my left ear is feeling strange again. It has been for a couple of days, so no doubt I will be heading back to the doctor soon for my ears. Oh goody.

Headaches: I have never been a sufferer of headaches. Like most people, now and then I would get one. The headaches I have suffered since Ms Menopause arrived have been horrible. I know that we lose oestrogen at this time and it does affect the brain. The worst of them was when I was on HRT. At times the pain was unbearable. I then started to depend on Panadol, which I have never done before. I still get headaches, but thank god, not as constant or as harsh since I have been off HRT.

Chapter 12

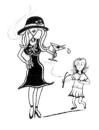

OH, OKAAY!

These are the comments that have been made to me since this stage of my life began. There is no disrespect aimed at any of these women, I have just found all of these comments quite interesting. A few I spoke to thought we get more hormones with menopause. Many women have no idea what happens. These are intelligent, independent women. Some have raised families and some have not. It made me realise that it wasn't just me, as at one stage I had been pondering, thinking maybe there had been a big announcement or women had been educated, and I just missed it.

I had a chat to a lovely woman who was in her early sixties who told me that not every woman goes through the change, and she was one of them. To be respectful, all I could mumble was, "I thought every woman in the world will deal with menopause." I would agree with her and this comment if the woman was a transvestite, a cross dresser, or even a transgender. I would also agree with her if she had had both her ovaries surgically removed before she reached puberty, but all I was hearing in my head as I walked away from her were: crickets! Knowing what I know now, many women meet Ms Menopause in their sixties - I hope that she is okay.

No disrespect to cross dressers, transvestites or transgenders by the way. You have a right to be happy in your skin just like everybody else. I must admit though, I just get a, well, a l-i-t-t-l-e jealous sometimes when you look fabulous and beautiful and lots better than me, and I am the real deal. Not fair!

Another woman I know started to tell me that menopause had not even bothered her, then said her husband had thought she had turned into a witch and that she has now been on her HRT for eleven years. I asked her what would happen if she went off HRT. She said she would suffer with depression. A friend of hers went off HRT because of side effects and is now having to deal with depression. So damned if you do, and damned if you don't.

I spoke to a friend who is in her seventies. She told me that her experience with it wasn't too bad, but went on to tell me that a number of her friends, younger and older, are having quite a terrible time with it, and some are still dealing with it in their seventies. I questioned her on why she thought that Ms Menopause was not put more in the spot light. This was her response: "It's a bit like childbirth, why scare the heck out of women before it happens?"

As I walked away, for one small moment I did think it was quite a logical statement, but faster than they can split an atom I thought, no! Childbirth is most often a choice. Our hormones go bonkers during and after pregnancy but eventually everything goes back to normal. Menopause is not a choice. Every woman will lose hormones that she will never get back. The loss of these hormones plays havoc on an otherwise healthy woman. Women need to know what they could be facing when Ms Menopause knocks.

Now it used to baffle me why it is called "The Change". I would correct people who used that term with me and inform them, "I am going through menopause."

Now, I personally am not dealing with all the symptoms I am about to list, but stay with me. Women can get the menopausal moustache, hair growth on chins, bald patches on heads, bloating in the stomach region. I am not able to multi-task anymore. I can only concentrate on one thing at a time due to memory loss and brain fog. I get horrible fatigue. I can't do much housework, cooking or shopping. I have to keep my fingernails short so that I don't scratch the hell out of myself. I have not been able to wear makeup for a long time as it irritates my skin and, what the hell, let's also add in the fact that I am short.

Oh my gawd! Short, bald, with a moustache, beard and beer gut. I don't do much around the house, and can only do one thing at a time. Oh, okay! I get "The Change" now!

A note to all those wonderful men who have been doing their fair share in the home. Keep going!

Chapter 13

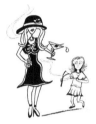

DOCTORS, AND ONE YIKES

My doctor was on holiday and I needed to get a new script, so I went and saw another doctor. I asked this doctor what the symptoms of menopause are as it was early days for me and I was quite clueless. The doctor looked at me and in all seriousness said, "You get a dry vagina." That was it. He looked at me, I looked at him, I slowly picked up the script and mumbled, "Thank you," and backed out of his office thinking, "He could have been lickin' his lips as he said it!"

Out of all the symptoms that he could have told me about, that was the only one he came up with. Yeah, no wonder women are hesitant to talk to their doctors. Thanks God for giving me a fabulous and respectful doctor. I didn't tell my doctor about this "frozen moment in time" but I did inform him that he was NEVER, EVER, EVER allowed to go on holiday again.

If I knew then what I know now I would have said something to him regarding his lack of respect, or I might have reported him, not to get him in trouble, but to make him aware that he needs a lot of educating on menopause and people skills. It is unacceptable and unethical. At one point I stumbled upon the following:

"Depending upon the perspective one has about "The Change of Life", it can be viewed as a positive or negative."

Here we go again. So you are trying to tell me that depending on the perspective I have when dealing with menopause, that that is going to determine whether I will suffer or not? Give me a break. Hey, maybe if I had just smiled and sung "Always look on the bright side of life" I would not have lost hormones at all, or even better, I may not have gone through menopause at all!

There is no positive to Ms Menopause when a woman is suffering with symptoms, no matter how positive or negative her perspective is. And don't even get me started on the site I again stumbled onto that said, "Menopause is the time to release your Inner Goddess." Look, good on them if that is how they feel. I am happy for you. Maybe the woman who sails through menopause also feels this way, but for me, ain't no self inner goddess releasing herself here. Just my inner, older self, trying to release herself, fifty years too early, trying to make me morph into that male version of myself!

I was at a chemist trying to work out the best Vitamin D supplement for me when a lady started to chat to me about what she takes. Of course we ended up having a talk about menopause. This is the conversation we had:

ME: How was menopause for you?

LADY: I always remember being terribly unwell through it.

ME: So how did you know you were through it?

LADY: I don't know, I just remember once I got through it I was old. I am eighty-four now.

Yikes, sorry I asked!

I thought that was the end of the conversation, but just before she walked away with her huge bag of medical needs, she came over and gently held my wrist. At that moment I got visions of fine china teacups and cucumber sandwiches. This beautiful lady then leaned in and said to me, "It also affects your sex life. You won't feel up to having sex." I replied, "Thank you, but I am single, thank God, so I don't have to worry about that extra stress at the moment."

What a wonderful woman. Thank you. I enjoyed meeting you immensely. Oh and I had to stop taking the Vitamin D tablets as for some reason I had a reaction to them which I need to find an answer for.

Chapter 14

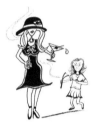

SICKO

This one wasn't originally going to get his own chapter, but after what I have read, a lot more needs to be said about this man. To be truthful, I don't really want to put this creep anywhere, but he needs to be mentioned. This is a condensed version. Here goes:

Who the hell is Sigmund Freud? I had heard of him, but his name was popping up all over the place in my research about Ms Menopause. This is what I originally read about him:

> He had a male-dominated theory of human development, which, unfortunately, set the foundation for the theory of menopause.

> Sigmund based the meaning of a woman's life, or her power, on her ability or inability to bear children, so the post-menopausal woman's life fundamentally has no purpose, she, becomes invisible.

Give me a break! As far as I am concerned he is just another man in the 1800s to early 1900s who had a bit of power and the gift of the gab, who thought and was allowed to do and say, whatever he pleased. Another one of those men determining our worth, and deciding how we feel. Off I went to research this man. I certainly hope the medical community is not guided by this sicko!

Sigmund Freud, Born 1856 - Died 1939. He was the father of psychoanalysis, a physiologist, a medical doctor, and a psychologist. He wrote a piece on "Infantile Sexuality" which took the innocence of a child away. He also wrote a piece on the abuse of children in Vienna. His paper suggested that the abuse was the child's fault and desire. This man also offered up another theory on the same subject, which was met with anger and disgust, and which he then quickly withdrew. Thank God those who stood up against him did so. These brave people put the safety, wellbeing and best interests of children first. I personally think he himself had underlying "desires", and if he lived today, me thinketh he would be in jail, where he belonged.

Why did I write this? It was too important not to. Firstly, the obvious disregard for women. The theory on post-menopausal women was only his thoughts. To say a woman has no purpose and becomes invisible was based on what may I ask? It was his personal opinion, nothing more, nothing less. No great theory, just some geezer living in his male dominated century.

Why did it become the foundation for the Theory of Menopause? I am sorry. I feel like laughing, it is so absurd and ridiculous to think he was a forefather of the medical world. His theory of human development makes no sense. Oh I am so sorry, but am I missing something here? At least I am feeling a very small giggle gathering deep down from the absurdity of it all. "Having no purpose" isn't a natural human development. "Becoming invisible" is not a natural human development. Wouldn't each of these have to be taught human developments, that is, women would have to be taught, or socialised into believing, that they have no worth. He comes up with this stupid, male chauvinist thought, he turns this thought into a theory, it is published and discussed. And all of a sudden, post-menopausal women are treated as though they have no purpose and are made to feel they are invisible. Just because this bloke had a thought.

Secondly his disregard for the child was disgusting. I believe we all have a right to our own fantasies, but when those fantasies include children and taking the rights of any woman away, in any generation, that is when a person's fantasies and desires become a criminal offence in society. He was a bully and a sicko who chose to pick on those who were vulnerable and who could not defend themselves.

Did you know Sigmund was a cocaine user? Now before I go on, back then cocaine was used for its medicinal properties. Also, where do you think Coca-Cola got its name from? Yep, Coke's origin was cocaine and caffeine. I say origin but there are debates even today that are saying the "safe" part of the coca leaves that are still used in Coke today may not be as safe as assumed. I have seen many people drink Coke to the degree that they seem to be addicted to it, so maybe there is something to this debate. Don't sue me Coca-Cola, because if you have any thoughts along those lines you will have to get in line as Ms Menopause is already stripping me of all I am and all that I had!

Freud also advocated the use of cocaine for his patients and used it for a variety of purposes. When the addictive and harmful side effects became known, his medical reputation suffered. I find it interesting that this man who was so interested in thought patterns and human behaviour was advocating and using a drug that alters the above, which he would have been fully aware of being a user himself.

To ponder a painting painted by an artist who was drugged up to his eyeballs as he was painting it is one thing. For someone in the medical world, especially in the field he chose, to be using and also getting his patients to use a drug that alters their thought patterns and behaviour is another thing. He was dealing with lives. They say he was interested in its antidepressant effects. Oh really? Oh ok.

Dr Carl Jung, who Sigmund originally saw as his successor, also distanced himself from Freud. In a movie I watched about this creepy geezer - yes this movie came on TV in the middle of research into Freud - Dr Jung told his wife that every time he asked Freud a question, Freud would always answer it with sexual connotations. A rift developed between the two when Dr Jung started to veer away from Freud's beliefs on psychoanalysis.

Psychoanalysis: Method used where the patient is encouraged to talk freely about personal experiences, especially about early childhood and dreams.

Dr Jung felt that this method could reveal the cause of the patient's problems but it could not cure it. I reckon Sigmund was only in it to hear the juicy stories, he couldn't give a toss whether it cured the patient or not. And how much fun was Sigmund having when on cocaine and giving it to his patients? I was walking past a bookshop and saw a sign saying, "Three for $10." I actually thought they were small, good sized blank diaries, so I went in thinking I needed more blank paper to scribble my notes on. I looked down at the table and realized they were books of about 100 pages and guess which book was right there in front of me? Yeppo, it was Sigmund Freud's book, "Deviant Love." Am I surprised by the title? No. The front cover had a photo of a phallic flower on it. No surprise there, and it was translated by Shaun Whiteside. Why you would want to translate this rubbish into English is beyond me, but it has helped my research and given me more ammunition against Freud.

I want to know why his stupid and disgusting theories and his cocaine-fuelled ramblings have been allowed to spill over from his time into the 21st Century. It actually concerns me that I was able to buy this book from the bookstore. I am a big girl, I can look after myself, but his obvious disrespect for innocent children is a different battlefield all together.

I didn't want to spend my five bucks on buying this one book, but knew if I was going to mouth off I needed to know as much about him as I could. When I handed my money over I said to the woman, "I really can't stand this man, but I have to read up about him." Of course I then asked "Have you got any books on menopause?" This time they did, three in fact. A few months earlier I had gone in and asked a different sales assistant the same question and they had none.

I am finding it very hard to read this book and I know it is going to be a very long time before I fully read it, if I ever do, but I will give you three snippets of information from it:

He compared mothers to whores. He wrote about the child again. And he wrote:

> "Girls are more intelligent and livelier than boys at the same certain age, but because of their "pubic hair" women only invented plaiting and hair weaving and otherwise made almost no contributions to the discoveries and inventions in the history of civilization."

I can't read this whole book, what I have read makes me sick and infuriates me, but I will be keeping it as ammunition if any one tries to defend him to me. Today Sigmund Freud would be considered a paedophile, a drug addict, a sexual deviant and a male chauvinist pig. It got me thinking about female inventors in history, and here is a list of some women and their inventions in alphabetical order in his lifetime from 1856-1939:

Beehive	Thiphena Hornbrook	1861
Brassiere	Mary Phelps Jacob	1913
Cabinet Bed	Sarah Goode	1885
Car Heater	Margaret Wilcox	1893
Cooking Stove	Elizabeth Hawk	1867
Dam & Reservoir Construction	Harriot Strong	1887

Dishwasher	Josephine Cochran	1872
Electric Hot Water Heater	Ida Forbes	1917
Fire Escape	Anna Connelly	1887
Globes	Ellen Fitz	1875
Improved Locomotive Wheels	Mary Jane Montgomery	1864
Life Raft	Maria Beaseley	1882
Locomotive Chimney	Mary Walton	1879
Medical Syringe	Letita Geer	1899
Oil Burner	Amanda Jones	1880
Refrigerator Cooling System	Florence Parpart	1914
Washing Machine	Margaret Colvin	1871

There are so many that I haven't mentioned them all. However I need to mention one more that came later:

Barbie Doll	Ruth Handler	1959

The reasons for this add-in will become clear shortly.

Throughout time it has always been men doing the prodding, thinking, talking, snipping and poking for or of women. For too long men have determined a woman's worth. I don't believe any man (or woman) has any right to hold back any information in regard to a woman's body or mind. Regardless of what we do or do not know, we will meet Ms Menopause. We will still lose our hormones and deal with the symptoms. Do they think we don't go through menopause because they have decided to put an invisible blanket over it? A woman needs, and has a right to, this information. Knowledge is power, knowing the facts will give you the power to deal with it on your terms, and not on the terms of the medical community or society in general.

Chapter 15

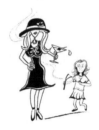

STOP PRESS! HELLO ADRENAL GLANDS

I was researching Ms Menopause to find some logic to her. I was looking at three sites and as I read each of them I noticed that the adrenal glands were being mentioned, not in detail, just in regard to how our glands and hormones rely on and interact with each other. After seeing it for the third time I knew I had to have a look into these adrenal glands. Well pop that bottle of champagne - for those who can still drink - hmm. I must admit it put a smile on my face. I actually did a wee five-second jig in my lounge room - that's the most dancing I have done since you know who turned up. I miss dancing!

This is what I discovered:

Christine Northrup MD spoke of adrenal exhaustion and what we need to know about it in regard to menopause. She wrote:

> The adrenal glands are your body's primary shock absorbers. These two little thumb sized glands sitting on top of your kidneys produce

hormones including adrenalin, cortisol and DHE allowing us to get on with our daily life in a healthy and flexible way.

Adrenalin is commonly thought of as the "flight or fight hormone". This is produced when something is (or you think it is) threatening you. It makes your heart pound and your blood rush to your heart and large muscle groups. Basically it prepares you for battle.

Cortisol increases your appetite and energy level and tones down your immune systems allergic inflammatory response. This helps the body to resist the stressful effects of infection, trauma, temperature extremes and helps us to maintain stable emotions.

DHE is an androgen that is produced by both the adrenal glands and ovaries. DHE helps to neutralize the cortisol's immune-suppressant effect and helps resistance to disease. It also aids to protect and increase bone density and guards cardiovascular health by keeping "bad "cholesterol levels under control, also providing vitality and energy etc. It is the main ingredient the body uses to manufacture testosterone.

Guess who adrenal gland rings when it's depleted? Progesterone! The adrenal glands borrow - actually take as they don't give back - from progesterone which is completely depleted to zero percent through dealing with Ms Menopause. When we lose estrogen through menopause, it is the adrenal gland's job, if healthy, to kick in and start producing estrogen. Yes! Apparently adrenal glands can make estrogen!

I also want to add the following, again please stay with me here. It is from the "Discovery - Fit and Healthy" website:

The adrenal glands are needed to respond to stress. It was designed to deal with our stress in small spurts. Thousands of years ago our stress responses were not asked to last days or months. If we encountered a lion, we would need to fight the lion, flee from it or be eaten by it. This type of stress would have been decided in a matter of seconds or minutes.

This is much different to the daily attacks that a bad boss, a terrible trip, a bad relationship or a chronic illness could bring. While our minds know that a bad boss at work does not threaten our lives, from the neck down, the adrenal glands and the other organs respond by hearing the same instinctive claims.

So the stress we may encounter day in and day out at work and in the other areas of our lives would be sending the message, "LION!" Faint - oops, I mean run! The body can run from the lion for a very short distance, but it was not made to outrun the lion every hour of the day.

I sat down and compared all the menopause symptoms to the exhausted adrenal gland symptoms. You will be very surprised.

Menopause Symptoms	Exhausted Adrenal Glands
period irregularities	period irregularities
excessive fatigue	fatigue debilitating
cravings for sweets	craving sweets
memory loss	memory problems
headaches	headaches
weight gain	weight gain
mood swings	mood swings
depression	depression
irritability	irritability
loss of sex drive	low sex drive
vaginal wall weakness	vaginal wall weakness
inability to deal with stress	can't deal with stress
sleep disturbance	sleep disturbance
dizziness	dizziness
increase in allergies	allergies worsen/inflammation
low libido	decline in libido
exacerbation symptoms to health issues	reduced resistance to existing health issue
fatty tissue in stomach	weight gain in stomach

hot flushes	hot flushes
bloating	swelling of stomach
weakness of the	weakness of the
immune system	immune system
insomnia	insomnia
internal shaking	disruption in tremor nervous system
digestive problems	indigestion
muscle weakness	muscle weakness
brain fog	thinking is foggy

Wow!

If a woman has adrenal fatigue, she tends to have more difficulty in menopause. Why are we not told this? A woman with healthy adrenal glands can still have a very horrible experience with Ms Menopause, but it makes the journey more debilitating if her adrenal glands are fatigued. When a woman is struggling to the extent that she is unable to function in the world or even in her home life, why isn't it suggested that her adrenal glands be checked?

The main problem for adrenal gland fatigue is stress. Too much stress that is pretty well constant can exhaust our adrenal glands. It could be financial worry, bad marriage or relationship, death of a loved one, lack of relaxation, overexertion, allergies, stresses at work, lack of sleep, poor eating habits, toxins, infections, fear, and more. I reckon these stress triggers apply to every person in the world. For the menopausal woman though, the debilitating effect of this only occurs due to Ms Menopause showing up and stealing those hormones.

If exhausted, fatigued adrenal glands are left untreated, unrelated conditions such as asthma, respiratory infections, allergies, frequent colds, rhinitis, chronic fatigue syndrome, adult on-set diabetes, auto immune disorders and so on can appear.

So let's sum up a little here. I now know that the adrenal glands sit - more like sloth - on top of our kidneys and that they are thumb size. The pain that felt like a "knuckling" feeling was in my lower back but I thought it was my kidneys. Now look at your thumbs, now look at your knuckles. Same size eh! A big symptom for adrenal gland exhaustion is craving salt. I was also craving salt!

Even when I was admitted to hospital in July 2012 and told the doctor about craving salt and the knuckling feeling in my lower back, not once were the adrenal glands mentioned. Why not? In fairness to the doctor, and let it be mentioned she was lovely, the adrenal glands can read as normal in a blood test even though they might be depleted. But, in fairness to me, why wasn't the craving for salt and the knuckling sensation investigated a bit further? I am not saying that I have adrenal gland fatigue, but I personally think it is worth investigating.

I marched into my next appointment with all this new information in hand. I had the appointment booked as I was getting results of a pelvic ultrasound, abdominal ultrasound, a pap smear test and to have my fun monthly desensitization...zzzzzz. Wake up! All tests came back fine, except for a slightly fatty liver and a fatty pancreas. For now those can sit on the backburner with, "Why is my stomach feeling heavy at times and as if it's about to fall," until I get the adrenal glands sorted. Oh they couldn't find my right ovary, it was suggested it has shrivelled up and considering they are only approximately 3cm in size, well not a big loss. Yay, one down, one to go.

I spoke to my doctor about what I had experienced and showed him the comparison of menopause symptoms versus the fatigued adrenal glands symptoms. The comparison even surprised him. I requested to get my adrenal glands checked so off I went to pathology to collect a container to collect my wee in for twenty-four hours.

When I saw the container, well put it this way, do you remember those big glass bottles of wine, lovingly called "goonies" that some of us drank in our younger days just because they were cheap? Yeppo, a bit like that but plastic, squarer and bigger and hell yeah, it even came with its own funnel. The only thing that came out of my mouth when I saw that container was, "Does that come in a bag?" Indeed it did, thank God. There was no way I was going to carry that thing, in all it's glory, hanging out and swinging in the wind, back to the car. I have a bit more dignity at this age, not like when I was eighteen, when the old goonie was passed around for all to see. So la la la... la la la... la la la la laaaaaa. Twenty-four hours have passed, it is back in the bag to go back to the pathologist, my work here is done.

The nurse I usually deal with for blood tests was back. I handed her the bag and paperwork. She said, "This is a different one," then reached for the "Tests Manual," but I told her it was not in there and that the previous nurse had to ring somewhere and speak to the Duty Scientist as she wasn't sure whether I was to take home the normal container or the acid container. I needed the normal container. So that was fixed, the nurse then looked down at the paperwork and said, "I wonder what this is for?" Had I walked out of the room without knowing it? I told her how I found that maybe the adrenal glands, if not healthy, could be adding to the suffering of a woman dealing with menopause.

This is the rest of the conversation:

Nurse: Oh yes! ok... [Said in a way that suggested she already knew that!]

Me: So you already knew that?

Nurse: Oh, there are lots of things that can go wrong in regard to menopause, we just feel it's not a good idea to bombard women with too much. They might get tests done, then when the tests come back ok, they think, "Oh why did I bother doing that?"

Me: Well I reckon a woman would be able to determine how she is travelling throughout menopause and suffer less than is needed if she knew other factors could be contributing to her struggle.

I was shocked. I will tell you when I am feeling bombarded with too much information. Geez almighty!

I was told by both of the pathology nurses that my results would be back in two days. Ok, one week has passed. Two weeks have passed, now this is getting ri-dic-u-lous!

After many calls back and forth between myself, the doctor and the nurse, I found out that these tests have to go to New South Wales as Queensland does not have the testing equipment.

So, this was put in for testing on the 5th of December. I found out today, the 20th of December, about my urine having a nice trip away to NSW. It is a few days away from Christmas, so I am putting all that away to enjoy this wonderful celebration as best as my health will allow, with my family and friends.

Now it's turning into an epic journey. Today is the 28th of December, one day before I turn fifty-two. A call comes through from the pathology nurse, a different one - so this makes it three pathology nurses I have dealt with - to advise me that the urine test has to be done again as I was given the wrong container. I was given the normal container when I should have been given the "acid" one. Well talking about "acid," I must admit I really did want to turn into an acid-tongued cow for a moment. You have to be joking!

I wasn't angry with the nurse, why would I be, even though they abide by a secret code in their medical world when it comes to Ms Menopause. I did tell her that it did not make sense as the other nurse had checked with the duty scientist about the correct container I needed. When this nurse rang me back, after my questioning it, she went and double-checked it for me. The story changed, apparently the doctor had requested the wrong test for me. So wrong container or wrong test? Will I ever know? I am guessing not. After twenty-three days, I get told this? It doesn't ring right to me. As said to the nurse, I am not just being tested to see if I have a common cold, this test is

94

for my adrenal glands. Bad luck if I was dying eh. I do the twenty-four hour "wee" thing again on the 30th of December, I will hand it in back in on the 31st of December. I started trying to get my adrenal glands checked in 2012, I will get my results in 2013. This time I have been advised that the results will be back in a week. I hope this delay and the mucking around does not make my health problems bigger than they already are, because this time I will make a gigantic noise about it.

It is shameful that this has turned into such a trial. I want my adrenal glands checked medical world. I am paying for it to be done. I am not even sure if my adrenal glands will be fatigued, but it is my right to get them checked. It took you twenty-three days to tell me all this, how about trying the truth? It really doesn't make sense to me considering I have been told that this new test will take a week for the results. Oi, medical world that is S-E-V-E-N days! So how did it take twenty-three days to tell me about the error? The amount of time it took you to let someone know about this mess may, for some, be the difference between having to be medicated for life or not. And, let's not forget that overall its has taken five weeks, FIVE WEEKS, to get the results of my adrenal gland test which, apparently, should have taken a week.

The extra four weeks it has taken could mean the difference between life and death for some. I am not angry with my doctor. I am angry that it took you twenty-three days to advise anyone! The way women are treated has to change big time in regard to menopause-related tests. So I will just wait now until the results come back, hopefully in this decade!

I have also just been advised by my doctor that steroids suppress the adrenal gland function. I hate steroids, always have, always will. I have hated my daughter having to take them in her younger life and I now hate the fact that I have had to use them, but unfortunately they are the only thing, or so I keep being advised by doctors, that apparently can save lives. That also was pretty evident when I went to hospital. I was sent home on steroids, and on the second trip when I was admitted, my steroids were upped to 50mg. I still hate them, I know they will create side effects, but right now I haven't a choice. Well, not a choice I have found yet, one thing at a time.

Chapter 16

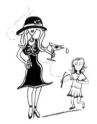

COINCIDENCE OR GUIDANCE?

Initially when I started scribbling notes onto any piece of paper I could find, I was doing it for myself. I had to understand what was happening to me. I never for one moment thought Ms Menopause was bigger than just estrogen, progesterone, mood swings and a hot flush here and there.

I had heard, somewhere, that we have adrenal glands in our body, oh so we have two of them. Oh ok. I just found out that insulin is actually a hormone too. What did I think insulin might be before? No idea! All I knew about it was that it had something to do with diabetes and it came in a syringe in liquid form.

I do know now that the body is quite a marvellous network of hormones, glands, organs etc. that are so finely tuned that if one is affected it causes a ripple effect right throughout the rest of the body. I look back now and I think, this is the book I was going to write even before I knew it. Ok you may think it sounds loopy, we all know now I believe in angels. I am not a believer in coincidence. As one very famous person once said, "Coincidence is God wearing a fake moustache and dark sunglasses," and I agree. So I personally believe the next two stories I am going to tell you, while we fill in time until my adrenal glands test results come back, is guidance. You, the reader, can draw your own conclusions.

As I have been writing, my daughter has been doing some typing for me as my energy levels are low most of the time. We have set it up on her laptop, it is portable and she can take it and print off drafts and type for me when required. When I have scribbled enough, I do some typing if I am up to it. When I am scribbling notes, I can have any noise around me, music, television and so on as it doesn't bother me. When I am typing, noise distracts me, so I have everything turned off.

I had settled down to do a bit of typing, when the laptop just turned itself off. It hadn't done this to me before. I checked that everything was plugged in, I turned it back on but could not find the programme we are using for our typing. I was quite annoyed as I really had some good energy to get some done and the daughter was out living her life and wasn't around to fix the problem for me. I kept thinking, "Let it go," as I have learnt even little, insignificant stresses seem bigger to me now.

I put the television on to help put my head somewhere else for a while to help me stay calm. Sounds dramatic, I know, but stress is really something I can't deal with. If I get upset or angry it affects my whole being and to be honest, it makes me feel like I am going crazy. I know I could crack in the blink of an eye when stress occurs, so I try and stay calm. This doesn't mean I don't stand up for myself or I don't use my voice anymore, I know the difference. This is coming from me who used to love the saying, "Don't sweat the small stuff," but always stood up for my rights. I feel that if I "lose it" I may not get back to me.

Anyway, the TV is on due to the laptop turning off. I was watching an overseas medical show where they were interviewing a woman in her mid-fifties about her illness. This woman had been very sick dealing with extreme fatigue, mood swings, lack of concentration and she was craving salt. I'm watching this thinking, "sounds familiar".

The woman didn't go to the doctor for a year, even when her skin started to get darker. The first doctor she saw told her that it was probably the drive to and from work that was causing her extreme fatigue. The second doctor she went to checked her blood pressure and told her it was a little high or low, I can't remember which one, but that was all he did. The third doctor told her that what she was dealing with was all in her head. What is wrong with these doctors? It was only when her son came home for holidays and saw how much his mum had deteriorated that he drove her back to the hospital and insisted there was something seriously wrong with her.

So the doctors started to do tests. They all showed that her adrenal glands were depleted and she had Addison's disease. Addison's disease means that your adrenal glands are stuffed. This woman now has to live on medications for the rest of her life.

To be fair, even with all these symptoms this woman didn't go to the doctor for a year. Her craving for salt was so extreme that she would eat cups full of rock salt and would add salt to her beer. The other main change was her skin colour which looks like an overdone, bad sun bed job. She should have gone to a doctor earlier so has to take some responsibility for the outcome of her health problems, but three doctors sent her home! Wake up to yourselves Medical Community! When we are telling you something is not right with our bodies or we just don't feel well, listen! We know our bodies. Even if that woman had gone to the doctor a lot sooner, she still would have been sent home by three doctors!

If anything changes in your body, make sure you get it checked, don't leave it. Definitely don't let any doctor tell you nothing is wrong. The adrenal glands are too important. If I was a doctor, I would have gone and found out what my knuckling feeling and craving for salt could have been, but it is only through the research I have done since

Ms Menopause arrived that I have learned of the link with the adrenal glands.

I am just so thankful that I am not dealing with Addison's disease. Well my skin colour hasn't changed, so I am assuming I'm not. With exhausted adrenal glands I will in time be able to heal and get them healthy again. This will allow me to only have to deal with the allergies caused by Ms Menopause, and to deal with just Ms Menopause herself. No wonder I have been feeling like I am dead, but am still breathing.

The daughter came home and there was no reason for the computer to do what it did. The programme was there for the typing. So I believe this was guidance. I was meant to see that programme about the adrenal glands. I reckon with all this adrenal gland stuff popping up all of a sudden, that if my tests come back normal, then I was meant to know this information so that I can alert other women to the adrenal glands. We will find out in 2013.

I was parking my car on the way to see my doctor with this new adrenal gland information. I had changed my appointment time as some days it takes forever just to get ready to see my doctor. Right in front of me was a group of eight women sitting at the hospital café chatting. They all looked to be between sixty and seventy years old. I sat there for a moment staring at them thinking, "Wow, I have never seen a group of women here before in the age group I need to talk to."

I was quite nervous as I wanted to go and have a quick chat with them before I headed in to my appointment. Then I thought bugger it, just do it. I went up to the women and asked them if I could ask them all a quick question. One of the women said "ONE question!" You know, it doesn't matter how much older we get there is always one in a group!

I explained to them in a minimum number of words that I was dealing with menopause and I was struggling, and I was wondering, in their experience with it, whether the adrenal glands had ever been mentioned.

The "one question" women shrieked, "Where did THAT come from?" You know lovee, I am nervous enough about approaching you all, stop adding to my nervousness! None of these women had heard about the link and were quite curious about it. I told them that I thought I had found why some women may be suffering even more through menopause and it is due to adrenal gland fatigue or exhaustion.

I had to head off to my appointment, but they said if they were still there when I came out, they wanted me to come back and tell them more and also let them know what the doctor said. Going by the empty cups of coffee and empty plates, it looked as though they had been there for a while.

Unfortunately I had a wait before I got in to see my doctor. After seeing him I had to walk over to the pathology office to collect my container, so by the time I got back to my car the "girls" were gone. I would have loved to have sat with them and chatted about their own experiences. I would have pulled up a seat and sat right next to the "one question" woman, because even though she added to my nervousness, I reckon she would have had a lot to say.

So, coincidence or guidance? I say guidance. I believe the laptop was meant to turn off for me to see the show on TV regarding the adrenal glands, and I believe I was meant to change my appointment time so that I could catch those women. Even though I didn't get to chat to them after, their response was enough to let me know that I wasn't alone in being kept in the dark on Ms Menopause.

I am looking forward to getting my results back. If my adrenal glands are ok I will be a little surprised, but happy. I feel good in knowing I stumbled on this link, it at least alerts women to the fact that with adrenal fatigue it can add to a woman's suffering when they are dealing with menopause.

Chapter 17

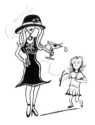

Q&A

Iam finding that with more knowledge, a lot more questions turn up too, which is a good thing. So here are the questions so far that I have put to my doctor, and the answers I have received. My doctor has a medical student with him at the moment, so he gave the student the questions and my doctor checked it before he returned them to me. I actually thought that was a great idea. Get this medical student a little bit educated about Ms Menopause before he even takes his place in the Medical World. New generations of doctors will hopefully bring new hope for menopausal women. Well it sounds promising.

My doctor also commented to me when he handed the answers back that he was quite impressed with my questions and that I knew my stuff regarding menopause. I told him that my learning about her and investigating her is purely and simply for my own survival, the survival of my daughter and hopefully many more women. But thank you my wonderful doctor for the compliment, it was appreciated.

Now I need it to be said, my doctor didn't agree with all the answers the medical student gave. After each answer there is an NB: which talks a bit more about the answers. I want to give you the answers exactly as the medical student answered them. Also I want to say thank you him for actually putting the time and effort he did into answering them.

Q: If HRT has estrogen and progesterone in it, why the need to add ten days of progesterone into the mix? Isn't this like double dosing, and have all HRTs got the two hormones in them?

A: Not all HRT regimens involve both estrogen and progesterone, but in general, both are involved. HRT regimens are designed to mimic a normal ovarian hormone cycle. As such, a base level of estrogen and progesterone are established, after which a ten-day progesterone dosage is administered to stimulate the normal progesterone increase in the pre-menopausal cycle.

NB: I am assuming here that the comment "In general, both are involved" basically means most HRT treatments have both hormones.

Q: If this is so, isn't this dangerous to a woman's health, putting too much synthetic progesterone in our bodies whilst on HRT?

A: Estrogen and progesterone levels are monitored and carefully tailored to what your body requires. That said, there are, indeed, risks involved with HRT therapy. This includes, but is not limited to, an increased risk of heart disease, strokes, emboli (a blood clot, piece of fatty deposit, air bubble or another object that has been carried in the bloodstream that can cause a blockage to a vessel), breast cancer, and endometrial cancer.

NB: How can a woman get her estrogen and progesterone monitored so that if she chooses to use HRT, it will be carefully tailor made to suit her body? As it stands now these HRT's are standard off the shelf ones, so they are not tailored to a woman's individual needs. From what I know none of the HRT products are anywhere close to being tailor made to a woman's individual needs. They are, I believe, very tailor made to make huge profits.

Q: Too much estrogen causes bloating. HRT causes excessive bloating, so does this mean the excess bloating caused by HRT is really due to too much estrogen being put into our bodies due to HRT?

A: It is true that estrogen may, indeed, cause bloating. This is noticed in both the peri-menopausal period (the period right before menopause) where estrogen levels are high and in certain hormone replacement therapy regimens. Additionally, bloating is observed in women undergoing menopause as well where estrogen levels may not be that high. In other words, bloating is a very non-specific symptom and while it is a common side effect of HRT, it does not necessarily mean that estrogen is the main culprit for the individual experiencing the symptom.

NB: When my doctor and I read the comment "bloating is a very non-specific symptom" we both said, "Don't agree with that," in unison. My doctor underlined it and put a question mark on it. I have experienced extreme bloating whilst on HRT and I reckon it was due to estrogen dominance. I still deal with bloating and very uncomfortable moments simply due to symptoms of menopause. Bloating is a very specific symptom of menopause regardless of whether you are doing HRT or not. I did think that maybe the comment was made in the context of meaning that we can get bloating from too much estrogen and from not enough estrogen, so really there is not one specific reason for this symptom.

Q: If we keep approx 40% of our estrogen and we lose all of our progesterone through menopause shouldn't we be looking at progesterone as being the main hormone that needs replacing, not estrogen?

A: A good number of the symptoms, such as hot flushes, are caused by the decrease of estrogen. Furthermore, a balance between the amount of progesterone and estrogen must be maintained if HRT is being considered. This is because progesterone affects the levels of estrogen and vice versa.

NB: Sounds good, but I feel you contradict yourself when further on you answer the question "Can I live without progesterone in my body?"

Q: Do we lose testosterone throughout menopause? If we do what does that do to us?

A: Production of testosterone declines gradually with age, so it isn't an abrupt loss of the hormone, as in the case of estrogen and progesterone. Decreased testosterone may be responsible for diminished libido, reduced energy, and an increased chance of osteoporosis, but more studies need to be done to establish the complete effects.

NB: Testosterone must decline faster in menopausal women for the symptoms above to appear. It is produced in a small amount in women. It is made by other hormones which are steroid hormones produced by the adrenal glands.

Q: I have heard that we can buy a natural progesterone cream. This is a part of the BHRT - Bio Identical Hormone Replacement Therapy. Any thoughts on that or do you know where I can get it from? Why haven't you offered me natural progesterone cream as an option or advised me of the BHRT option?

A: Currently, the evidence for a natural progesterone cream is inconclusive. This is, in part, due to the complex nature of progesterone as well as the lack of consistent results about its positive and negative effects within the scientific community. As such, I would recommend adhering to HRT. Natural progesterone is available currently with a prescription.

NB: Dr John Lee (you will learn more about this man later in this book) stood up to the Medical Community in regard to the dangers of HRT. He also pioneered the natural, yam based progesterone cream and studies showed it was alleviating woman's suffering and symptoms in a safer way than HRT. I am not saying that the natural progesterone or even natural estrogen is the answer for every woman, but I am saying that it gives all women a safer option than HRT. The comment, "I would recommend adhering to HRT," was a surprise. My doctor underlined the comment and wrote, "I don't agree." After I read it I got scared; been there, done that, never again. Of course a woman has the right to deal with menopause in her own way, but I feel natural is the safer and better way to go. I also do not think the comment on the scientific community holds any weight. The scientific community is tossing HRT at women when they are fully aware of the negative and dangerous effect it is having on them.

Q: At what stage through menopause does my estrogen level out? How long does it take to lose all of our progesterone?

A: This depends on your body. It can last five years or more. It starts from the first onset of menopause.

NB: I agree with this, but I would emphasis "or more." Once this process is done we still live with symptoms. I know women who are dealing with hot flushes in their seventies.

Q: Can I live without progesterone in my body?

A: Yes, after menopause women generally have little or no progesterone being produced in their bodies. Progesterone's main functions are related to reproduction, such as preparing the uterus for implantation of a foetus. However, progesterone does have some minor effects related to gum health and memory. Overall, aside from its effects on reproduction, the loss of progesterone does not have any other major effects on the body.

NB: Not too keen on this answer. This is the answer in which I feel you contradicted yourself. In a previous answer you stated, "progesterone affects the levels of estrogen and vice versa". My doctor didn't agree with this answer either as he stated that progesterone affects the levels of estrogen as well.

In fairness though maybe I should have worded it as follows; "I know we can be alive without progesterone in our body, but will a lack of it affect my quality of life?" I do not agree that "the loss of progesterone does not have any other major effects on the body." Progesterone production starts to decrease in our forties. Throughout menopause the low levels of progesterone causes symptoms such as mood swings, irritability, weight gain, depression and osteoporosis. Dr Lee showed through testing, that the use of natural progesterone relieves symptoms of hot flushes, dry eyes, night sweats, insomnia, bloating, irritability, gallbladder problems, hair loss, sore breasts and more. A study of bone density tests on Dr John Lee's menopausal patients who were trialing natural yam based progesterone cream, did indeed show significant bone density increase.

Q: When my estrogen levels out, will my allergy rate go down faster? What is blocking my allergy rate from going down faster?

A: A recent study by Bonds and Midoro-Horiuti in the United States shows that estrogen may have a link with specific allergies, such as asthma. It is difficult, however, to say how a more optimal estrogen level will affect your allergies at this point, as oestrogen's role in allergic disease remains complex.

NB: Great answer and very interesting.

Q: Do you think you can have more pink and white jelly beans in your jar next time I come in sobbing as they are my favourite?

A: My doctor and I discussed this one firstly and together, as we know it is the important question. My doctor had a laugh and then drew a smiley face as his answer. So that is a big thumbs up. My doctor also pointed out that I don't have to be sobbing to score more jellybeans if I want some. Yay! Thanks Doc.

NB: I have also noticed your jelly beans are the good quality glucose jelly beans bought from a chemist, not the cheap ones bought from a supermarket. I am impressed.

Not a bad effort for a medical student. Again the time and effort he put into answering these questions was appreciated even if we were not on the same page with a few of his answers. I know I still need to find out about tailor made HRT, so I will get back to you on that one but what I know at this point is only BHRT, the natural hormone therapy, that can be tailor made.

Chapter 18

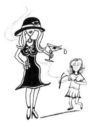

HELLO AND HAPPY
NEW YEAR 2013!

Well here I am in a New Year and the struggle continues. I had my sixth desensitization needle on the 3rd of January 2013, and two days later I was swollen and puffy, much more than an average day; it was quite disheartening. It felt like I had taken 1000 steps backwards. Normally I don't have a reaction to these needles, but on the odd occasion I have felt a bit dizzy at the medical centre. However I am not allowed to leave for twenty minutes after, so these few reactions are caught at the doctors, and the nurse monitors me for a moment. The dizziness doesn't normally last long.

My skin usually goes a bit strange after the injection, which is to be expected, but this time the reaction was a lot worse. I still have to count my blessings, I heard that a girl who also has these needles has such a bad reaction to it that they have to have an adrenal needle on hand in case they have to jab her with it. Poor pet. My Doctor is on three weeks holiday now. Yes! I was very diplomatic and wished him a happy holiday. So I will ask him about the harsher reaction when he gets back. I have had to up my steroids; even 1mg makes a big difference.

I also had six monthly blood tests done. I rang on Monday the 7th of January for results. My adrenal glands show normal and my allergy rate is down from 22300 to 18600.

I know I should be happy about both the above results but for some reason I am not. Normally I am a positive person, but as silly as it sounds, the results just made me feel sad. Why? Firstly I knew I was in for the long haul but getting the results really "stuck it in my face". A bit like the Liverpool-Glasgow kiss - BANG!

I am very happy my adrenal glands show to be normal. I can't help being a little curious about this, but that is what the results show. They are real little suckers to get results for. Before my doctor went on holiday he said that we may have to do another test which involves putting dye in my body, which makes the adrenal glands glow. Oh goody. I think if my doctor says that the urine test I did is 100% confirmation that my adrenal glands are ok, I probably won't have any more testing done on them. But something has to explain the knuckling feeling and craving for salt. This thought just keeps niggling at me.

I am very happy that my allergy rate has come down. It is the first time a lower allergy reading has happened since 2010. It's just that after having had the five months of fortnightly desensitization injections plus the six months of monthly needles, I thought my allergy rate would be a lot lower than it is. I know, I know, it is a positive that it is down, but yeah, just made me feel sad to know this, even though I knew it was going to take time.

I think what also made me feel sad was that all this suffering I am going through is all caused by her, Ms Menopause. I was thinking if my adrenal glands are fatigued, I can heal them and that would take one "side dish" away, so it would ease my suffering, right? Well obviously it is all Ms Menopause who is stirring up my allergies. I know she also affects the adrenal glands, but I was just hoping I could tick at least one thing off my list of many ills.

In all that has been learned about the adrenal glands though, I was wondering if they had been or are, healing themselves. I had a talk to my mate about the results and she made a comment that was along the same lines as my thoughts, but I hadn't said it out loud as yet.

Symptoms of fatigued adrenal glands I feel I suffer with are:

- Waking up groggy: I know with insomnia most of us are going to wake up fatigued, hell, even when you are healthy just getting out of bed is a bit push and shove at times. This grogginess feels different though. To explain, it feels for me as if someone had slipped me some sort of drug without me knowing and I was left feeling really groggy when I finally woke up. I have watched enough movies to be able to imagine this!
- Craving salt.
- Increased menopausal symptoms such as depression, lack of energy, muscle weakness, decreased ability to handle stress, increased allergies to mention a few.

Looking at all these symptoms I reckon adrenal gland fatigue is a relative of Ms Menopause. The healing of the adrenal glands includes quite a holistic approach, such as removing certain stresses from your life and resting, so maybe?

To add more to the pot of ills, there has been a flu going around, my daughter and a few mates have had it or are just getting over it. My poor brother woke up with it a day before he was to go back to work after holidays. I woke up with it a couple of days ago with a sore throat, stuffed up nose and just feeling like crap! Another crap feeling I have to deal with. Fabulous.

It all sounds so doom and gloom, but hey! Happy New Year to me, what else has this year got for my mind, body and soul to have to deal with?

I am now going to have a chat with Ms Menopause. It is immature and contains the word f… often. To personify menopause allows me to have my say to her.

Ms Menopause: Happy New Year Daaaarling

Me: Get fecked!

Ms Menopause: (sniggering) Just morph into that short, round, bald male version of yourself and I can tick that off your "Ovaries twenty-three billion, one million, one hundred and ninety two thousand, and for file."

Me: Feck off, ok? Wait a minute! Ovaries twenty-three billion whatever file? What the heck is that?

Ms Menopause: You are just ovaries to me sweetheart, nothing more, nothing less. You can't beat me daaaarling, there has only been one female in the whole world who has beaten me. She still has the very oversized supple and firm breasts of a twenty year old, even though she's in her fifties, she has the waist size that starving models would die for. She still has beautiful collagen filled features, lovely blonde hair, not a grey in sight now or ever. The words bloating, old, insomnia and depression will never pass her lips. Why? Well look under her dress sweetheart. This doll called Barbie that got away from me came with no girly bits! No ovaries, no suffering! I can't stand her!

Me: What the…? Geez almighty. Just leave me alone! You have to be feckin jokin'!

Ms Menopause: We both know that will not be happening, you silly, silly ovary keeper.

I know my conversation was not an intelligent one, but it's good to know that a plastic doll is a thorn in Ms Menopause's side. Here I was thinking she was so untouchable in every way. I will take what I can with her so if this plastic doll upsets her, I'm in! Quick get those old Barbie dolls out of storage daughter and create a big circle around me with them. Throw in a bulb of garlic and a wooden cross just in case, there are so many twists and turns with Ms Menopause, she could turn herself into anything in the blink of an eye. Better to be prepared just in case! She is a scary bitch!

I had never been a big fan of Barbie, but of course this doll was a part of the daughter's young life. I always felt it was not a good idea that little girls might see her as being how they "should" be. You can't tell me that some of the girls that played with her weren't scared and felt a bit abnormal when they peeked under her dress. "Muuum there is something wrong with me!" "No darling you are normal, Barbie isn't!" Imagine the terror when boys played with Ken or GI Joe!

Now I wonder if the creator of Barbie did it on purpose as a revenge thing to Ms Menopause. If so, clever woman, Barbie is still going strong today and is a billion dollar business just like HRT! Hey, hang on! Please don't tell me there is a connection here. Aw bugger it, my brain is too tired to even contemplate it.

As my journey with Ms Menopause limped on and since I'd thought these writings needed to be turned into a book, I decided I wasn't going to read any other books on menopause. I wanted my book to be about my experience and what I have learnt from my very limited research, and so didn't want any other influences.

I do know of two books you can buy which are supposed to be really good. The first is called *The Silent Passage* by Gail Sheehy. Personally, from what I have learnt, I would have titled it, *The Loud Turbulent Storm Tunnel*. But hey, that's just me, it is her journey with menopause. It was written in the 1970s, a bit outdated I thought, but there is a revised copy of it. I actually did go to look for it once in the very early stages of my dealings with Ms Menopause, but when I asked the guy at the counter (who mind you was just sitting there reading a paper -

love yar job eh mate?) he let me know without checking, that it was out of stock as it was a very popular book. I walked away thinking, "You had no idea what that book was about." Looking back I am really glad that he couldn't give a damn and that I haven't got a copy of it. If you decide to give it a read, take in what you feel is right for you, then spit out the rest. Exactly what I would expect you to do with my book. I am just hoping though, that with my book there is more taking in and less spitting out.

The second book is called, *What Your Doctor May Not Tell You About Menopause* by Dr John Lee. I always thought this sounded interesting but kept away from it for the reasons just mentioned. Funnily enough though, some things are just meant to come to us. I have been reading blogs by women from all around the world who are trying to figure out and find answers to their own journey with Ms M. I still do it in this new year, it always make me realize I am not alone, but now, more importantly, it has made me realize that women everywhere are looking for answers to combat Ms Menopause. I stumbled across a linked site where women were talking about the allergies they are dealing with since Ms Menopause entered their lives.

One of these women, trying to help the others out, quoted some good stuff out of a book she had been reading, guess which book it was, yep, *What your Doctor may not tell you about Menopause* by Dr John Lee. The following is the extract from Dr John Lee's book that this woman shared on the site. She also stated that since Ms Menopause arrived, she suffers epileptic seizures. I will condense it down. But before I start, I know that Dr John Lee is going to answer some of the questions that I have already asked in the "I'm Confused" chapter, but I kept that section in as it really is important to get all the questions answered, especially the one in regard to those jelly beans!

This is in the perimenopause stage, the time that Ms Menopause is lurking but hasn't really made herself fully known yet. They say it is a term used by women to describe the time they first notice menopausal symptoms. What a crock of crap, again! In my research, women don't even know they are heading into menopause, the result of lack of education, let alone know the bloody name for the first stage of it. As for me, I say, "Oh there are three stages to Ms Menopause? Feckin Fabulous!"

Anyway, onto the extract from Dr John Lee's book:

> When you are going through this period you may develop estrogen dominance. This could cause the following: acceleration of the aging process, allergy symptoms including asthma, hives, rashes, auto-immune disorders like lupus and sinus conditions.

He goes on to name many of the symptoms I have listed in Chapter 4, but also adds increased blood clotting which increases the risk of strokes, magnesium deficiency, dry eyes and zinc deficiency.

To simplify what he says, the combined effects of losing more progesterone than estrogen is more than enough to put a woman into a state of estrogen dominance. Stress in this first stage of menopause causes estrogen dominance which then causes insomnia and anxiety, which calls on the adrenal glands, if healthy, to create more estrogen and therefore more estrogen dominance. Let us not forget that adrenal glands also pull on our progesterone. Clear as mud ladies and that is the simplified version. I am writing it and I am not even sure if I get it!

What he is saying is that the loss of estrogen is not the real problem. Dr John Lee says that the loss of progesterone is the real problem and the main hormone we girls should be replacing through menopause is progesterone not estrogen. And you know, it does make sense. We keep some oestrogen, just at a lower level, but we lose all of our progesterone through menopause. Where am I going with this? I am not sure yet, but I have more on this doctor. Virginia Hopkins writes this. Again I am going to condense it:

> John R. Lee, MD, was internationally acknowledged as a pioneer and an expert in the study and usage of natural progesterone and on the subject

of BHRT therapy for women. Dr Lee used transdermal progesterone, meaning being administered through the skin by cream or patch, in his clinical practice for nearly a decade, doing research that showed it can reverse osteoporosis.

Dr John R Lee also famously coined the term "oestrogen dominance," which means a relative lack of progesterone compared to oestrogen, causing a list of symptoms familiar to millions of women. In the early 1970's he began dealing with a lot of menopausal women with health complaints who were not able to use oestrogen because of a high cancer risk, heart disease, or diabetes for example. At the same time he attended a lecture by Raymond Peat PhD who claimed oestrogen was the wrong hormone to be giving menopausal women, and that what they really needed was progesterone.

Dr Lee started suggesting that his menopausal patients try and use a progesterone cream that was natural and to his amazement his patients were delighted with the results. They reported relief from menopausal symptoms such as hot flushes, night sweats, insomnia, dry eyes, bloating, irritability, gall bladder problems, hair loss, sore breasts and more.

As a result of this positive feedback, Dr Lee researched progesterone more in depth, from his local medical library and through communications with scientists around the world. He realized that progesterone had a positive effect on bone health. A few years of studying bone density tests on his patients showed that these women were gaining significant bone density and those with the worst bone density to begin with were particularity showing great results.

WELL HELLO, clearer now? I had heard of natural progesterone cream, I asked my doctor questions about it and now Dr Lee is saying that the transdermal progesterone is the answer to helping to get Ms Menopause if not out of our lives, at least off our backs.

I feel like a broken record, CD, download - just covering all generations - but why don't we know this? Why aren't our doctors advising us of this? Why is HRT the only thing tossed at us menopausal woman? I reckon, to be cynical, I won't be able to get it on a script and that it will cost an arm and a leg. Hey, the medical student said it IS available on script! I know I need to try it first, but I am already thinking, "I need to get this natural BHRT on the PBS (Pharmaceutical Benefit Scheme, the list of medications that are subsidised by the government.)

Natural, not synthetic, progesterone cream really works to alleviate the symptoms of oestrogen dominance and the symptoms of Ms Menopause in general. Conventional medicine has failed to address these concerns in a safe, effective manner. Women, for decades, have intuitively known they are being mistreated by the medical community when it comes to HRT. Oh and did I just see a look of fear on the face of Ms Menopause for the first time since 2010? She could be just mocking me, but I say, "Let's just wait and see daaarling!"

John R. Lee M.D. passed away unexpectedly on Friday 17th October 2003, from a heart attack. Dr Lee was known by millions of people as the doctor who pioneered the use of transdermal progesterone cream and hormones that are bio-identical. This doctor had the courage to stand up against the medical establishment's dangerous and misguided HRT treatments. Thank you Dr John Lee, may you rest in peace. It is just so encouraging that Dr John Lee had the courage to stand up and speak out about the dangers of HRT and to actually do something about it. I am but one woman standing up, how much harder would it have been for this wonderful man to stand up against all his peers. I thank you and salute you for standing up for the women everywhere.

Chapter 19

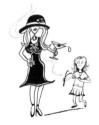

THESE DAYS TURNED OUT NOTHING LIKE I HAD PLANNED

As I learnt more about Ms Menopause and what she does to our bodies, I had very small, almost whispered, glimpses of understanding, but without any conviction or support to them, the medical world's decision, to toss women into the wilderness. A menopausal woman's body becomes like a labyrinth once we start losing our hormones and our bodies are affected in so many ways. But why does it have to turn into a labyrinth when it all stems back to just two hormones, estrogen and progesterone? After saying this, I will also say, "Not good enough Medical Community."

Imagine that Ms Menopause is standing there with a guitar and she plucks and snaps two strings, on purpose of course, as she knew you were really excited about playing some great music with it. So now the guitar is not working as well as it should because of the broken strings. Sure you can still get a bit of a tune out of it, but it won't give you the tunes you really want. Very much like our bodies during menopause, but, unfortunately in Ms Menopause's case, she won't be satisfied until all the bloody strings are snapped!

I was really excited about reaching my 50s. I always felt that they were going to be my best years. I obviously got that wrong. In saying best years though, I have had a wonderful life. Before settling down as a result of becoming a mum, I always said and felt that I had gypsy blood in me as I loved the freedom of moving around. I have had my share of happiness and sadness. I have travelled a little. I have danced in New Zealand and danced on a cruise ship and have danced in nearly all the states of this beautiful country of ours.

I have sung with the locals in Vila and flown down to Hobart just to see the best band, The Divinyls, in concert, which was fabulous. I have camped on Rottnest Island, slept on the beach and celebrated New Years Eve a few times in one night due to the time difference whilst living amongst the Quokkas. Scotland is the place I have always wanted to visit and explore since I was sixteen. I gave birth to my little baby who gave my life purpose, and I finally felt like I knew why I was here.

I have lost family members where the grief was unbearable; I have seen my daughter in pain to the extent where I wished I could have felt it for her. I lost my first love to a motorcycle accident at twenty-one years old. I have had great relationships and some not so great relationships. I have not always had that special person love me back the way I loved them, and vice versa. I have roared with laughter many times throughout my life, mostly with my daughter once she grew into her humour, fabulous! And have had many wonderful mates gatherings where we would chat, drink, laugh and at times cry.

I have seen some of the worlds' greatest bands and singers in concert.

I have not married yet, I was engaged once at twenty-five but just could not see it through to the end. Don't get me wrong, I personally am all for marriage. I am in awe of couples who do it and stay together for a lifetime. I did though, always find the concept of loving and actually liking one person for a lifetime, except for the wonderful family members and the daughter, a bit too big for me. I have always said, "Call me Elizabeth Taylor," because I too could have been married and divorced eight times, but it's all just a part of life isn't it? I have had the freedom of living in this wonderful country and doing the things I wanted. Through my travels I have met many fabulous people with many wonderful life stories. I have always felt the love and safety of my family, and that in itself is a blessing. But my greatest achievement, the most fulfilling and rewarding experience in my life, has and always will be my daughter. So, when all is said and done, I think I have done pretty damn well so far in this life.

My fifties for me always felt like, "Ok, I have paid my dues. I now will have more time for me and be a little more financially free. I am fifty. I will work where I want to work and be happy. No more jobs where I have to work just to bring in the dollars, all will now fit in with my lifestyle. I will do more travelling and finally get to roam Scotland. I will keep laughing and dancing until I can no more and if I meet that guy who loves me back at the same time I will, well maybe try, and make that commitment and marry him. If I never meet him, that too will be ok.

I will wear that bloody blue eye shadow if and when I want, even if it is not in fashion, oh wait a minute, that's right, I already do. I will dye my hair any colour I feel like, wow I do that already too. That tattoo of a cherry blossom branch on my wrist so it looks like a bracelet, I have been thinking of doing for a while, I may actually get it done. I will study two nights a week for that one course I have always been interested in and I will learn how to play the piano. I will be in the audience for the final of The Eurovision Song Competition one year. I will keep gathering the dollars, not for the materialistic gain, but for the freedom it gives to do what I want. I am not going back to my gypsy life though, as I know I would miss and fret for my family. I have a home, a box to put all my stuff in. I am happy, content, settled and healthy. Yeppo! That is the way my fifties originally felt, like they were going to be for me. Oh and I would finally win that million dollars on my bloody keno numbers!

Unfortunately Ms Menopause has pretty well snapped all of my strings and some days I feel there are not many strings left to snap. I have moments when I am absolutely in awe of how big Ms Menopause is and I think I am not capable or well enough to finish this book let alone get my health back on track and start actually living my fifties as I felt I was going to. On these days she wins!

For every turn I take on this learning path there is always something new or another twist in regard to her, and every day I wake up it seems there is another struggle to deal with, but every day a small part of me knows I am getting closer to being me again, and to being there for my family. How many times throughout my life have I said, "If you haven't got your health, you have nothing?" Who would have thought that I would one day arrive at a point where I'd be physically testing this worn out expression?

I have said many times in my past, "You can have a million dollars in your bank account, but it would be worthless if you haven't got your health to enjoy it." It will certainly take the stress away from worrying about money in ill health, but that isn't what life is about.

I still wake up swollen and groggy most days. I am tired. Most days I feel like I am not going to get there with my health. I still suffer with ear problems and headaches and symptoms of Ms Menopause. The depression still rears it's ugly head at times, I am tired of always being aware of my skin. My stomach still feels heavy, sore and as if it is dropping. I am still unable to pick up heavy things. I am still not able to deal with stress, but am managing it better nowadays. I look in my mirror and get a glimpse of how I thought I would look in my old age. That me in my old age isn't looking too bad but let's remember I am only fifty-two. I am in my middle age.

My friendships are disappearing except for a few, which is to be expected. I have not got much to say unless it is in relation to finding me again and my struggles with menopause, and I am not able to be there for my friends any more. I live, breathe and think Ms Menopause. I know this journey has put an enormous strain on my family and yet they still support me. At times I manage to do a shop, but it takes me hours to prepare for it and I still have moments of feeling overwhelmed by it all.

I still cannot deal with stress. This at times is starting to affect my relationship with my family. Yes this is about Ms Menopause and the effect she has on women, but the longer this journey goes on with her, the more I have realised that loved ones really suffer at times too. It isn't fair or easy on them. There are positives though, a little but very vital moment happens that helps to pull me back up and keep fighting.

My daughter and her friend prepared a lovely big healthy breakfast for all as they were heading out to The Big Day Out Music Festival. They knew it was going to be a long day of drinking, dancing and fun so the breakfast was prepared to help soak up those drinks and for energy.

My daughter then declared, "This will keep my adrenal glands happy too." Yes a proud and happy moment for a mother. So you have been listening to me daughter and your very own knowledge has started. My suffering all of a sudden didn't feel so big for that moment. My suffering also felt worthwhile in that moment. I love you because? As usual though, protecting your skin from the sun and drinking lots of water in between those drinks will also keep your mum happy.

I have been, knowingly, having to deal and live with Ms Menopause since 2010, today is 2013. She is one hell of a tough cookie. She and I still have a lot to sort out but I am still trying to put her in the back seat. 2013 has continued to bring other challenges, unfortunately, but before we do the gloom and doom stuff I would first like to dedicate the next page to my daughter and sing:

HAPPY BIRTHDAY TO YOU!
HAPPY BIRTHDAY TO YOU!
HAPPY 21ST BIRTHDAAAY
GAWJUZ DAAUGHTERRRR
HAPPY BIRTHDAY TO YOOOOOOU!

Wow, twenty-one years old. Is it the 23rd of January 2013 already? Wow didn't that go fast! In our relationship daughter, at times we have not understood each other, but you know what? I think that in itself is a healthy mother and daughter relationship. I love you and am very proud of you. You came and gave my life purpose and meaning. You have been and continue to be a wonderful daughter, I think I must have done something very special to be picked to be your mum. Oh and your sense of humour is priceless. You are one of the few people that can make me ROAR with laughter! I love you sweetheart. Mwah! Yar mamma. xxxooo

Now to the gloom and doom, but I still wouldn't want to live anywhere else in the world. We here in Australia have dealt with quite a lot of extreme weather conditions. In our little part of Australia, it was the floods. The water came in, around and under our house. I noticed that when it came to the clean up, I haven't got the stamina, strength or health to really get into it like I used to be able to before Ms Menopause moved in. We did all get there, but I can't say this time that I did my fair share of the cleaning up. Compared to many others, we came through it untouched really. So once again I count our blessings.

I am tired of it all. I have been off work now for seven months. Yes, it seems a long time, but when you are sick, time is strange. For some I am sure they dream of being a lady of leisure, but this period has not felt like leisure to me. Being sick is exhausting and expensive. It has been seven months of constant searching and battling and hoping to see me, once again, in my mirror and see me again in my eyes. I want to feel like me again. I want to be the mum, sister, best mate and mate I used to be. I see the strain it is putting on my family, and even though they have always supported me, it makes me so, so sad. I think I'm feeling a wee bit sorry for myself…

Right! Put your tissues away. A new day has arrived. Yesterday I was pathetic and ready to give up, today I am intending to keep fighting and writing. I have said to myself what I have always said to my daughter over the years when life sometimes gets tough, "Up you get, dust yourself off and get back into it." Last night I didn't sleep much at all but for the first time in a long time my lack of sleep was not the doing of Ms Menopause – yeah lovee, suck on them lemons!

It was because I couldn't stop thinking of the natural progesterone, and the more I thought about it, the more excited I felt.

Chapter 20

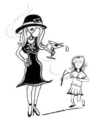

NATURAL PROGESTERONE

B HRT- Bio-identical Hormone Replacement Therapy. Hope has just walked in the door in the form of natural progesterone. So that's what hope looks like! I really needed to find this. It feels like the light at the end of the tunnel. I live to fight her for another day. My spirit is raised in knowing that natural progesterone may be a great help for me, for my daughter and many other women. I have a repeat moment of the wee jig I did when I found out the link between the adrenal glands.

I also know this new discovery may not be the answer to easing my suffering, but it is another product I can alert my daughter and others to in the hope it will at least help to ease some womens' suffering. I can't wait until my doctor comes back from holiday!

BHRT is plant based, more natural and safer. This can be tailor made to a woman's needs and there lies the answer to a question in the "I'm Confused" chapter.

HRT- Hormone Replacement Therapy, is synthetic based, has dangerous side effects and is a billion dollar business and cannot be tailor-made to a woman's needs.

I look forward to a discussion on this with my doctor, I think he has four days, seven hours, eleven minutes, and twenty-one seconds until he returns, hey but who is counting!

To be truthful, I was getting a bit lost in it all. With every turn and twist with Ms Menopause I was finding it was just getting too big for me. Was I giving up? Admitting defeat? Well maybe I was to a degree. At one stage I honestly thought that there is no winning your health back when you come up against Ms Menopause. She doesn't care how low she has to go to keep you down. Interesting how this new information about the natural progesterone was found just at the time I needed some hope.

This is what I reckon. If I had brought the book *What Your Doctor May Not Tell You About Menopause* by Dr John Lee at the beginning of my struggle with Ms Menopause, I know for sure I would be a lot healthier today, so I would never have even considered the need to write this book. So I reckon I wasn't meant to find this until the end of my journey, whenever that will be. How could I possibly talk and write and understand the issues and how debilitating menopause really is for women if I hadn't gone through it all myself? This coming from a woman who originally was planning the best menopause party to celebrate the arrival of it! Ha, you have to smile.

As bad as things can sometimes seem in life, and although we don't understand at the time why it is happening, up the track when we are through or on top of our difficulties, I have seen why that had to happen and usually the end result is a positive one. Of course there are things in life we can't control or fix which are heartbreaking and in some cases inevitable. Well death is inevitable for all of us. I personally would just prefer it to be later rather than sooner. I will be very, very ticked off if Ms Menopause is the cause of my demise.

I will tell you now, after I give my mum, my dad, my sister and my first love all big hugs, I will be knocking on the door of the main man upstairs, and asking, "What was *that*? Please explain." Or it could even be, "Oh my God, oh sorry God, what the…? You are a *woman!* Well then, what the hell were you thinking? Crash! Bang! Kapow!" Yeah! Definitely would be a bit of bitch slapping going on! Settle down people I believe God has a sense of humour. I am not scared to die, I just don't want to yet. I know it is not my call, but I want to have an old age and be healthy and be here for my loved ones and me.

I also have never had a problem with standing up against bullying or standing up for a good cause or for the underdog. Confrontation doesn't bother me if it helps to correct wrongs. So even though I cannot deal with stress at the moment, I still have my voice through these writings and it is a way to get out there how horrible this phase in a woman's life really can be when there is no need for it to be.

Today is two days away from seeing my doctor to get my seventh desensitization needle, and to chat about the new kid on the block, BHRT, the natural yam origin progesterone cream. I am excited! My twenty-one year old self is embarrassed that I am this excited, "Get a grip old woman!" Yes because at twenty-one, fifty-two is old. Me at fifty-two can't believe I am this excited over the progesterone cream, but I am! I yam what I yam and I yam very excited at the thought of the yam cream! I think, maybe, it's time for a rest. Hmmm.

Oh my God, thought to self: Did the universe give me a clue back then when I decided to name Chapter One: "I Yam What I Yam?" Being one that doesn't believe in coincidences, there is only one answer to that question. Why did I name it that? Well Popeye used to say, "I am what I am," or "I is what I is," or "I yam what I yam and that's all that I yam." I always liked the "I yam" and used to say it a bit when I was younger, mucking around with friends and maybe now and then in a past relationship. It just popped into my head for the title of chapter one. Well I'd better be on the right track with this yam stuff Universe, because I'm not re-writing pages and pages if it doesn't work! Oh geez!

Another matter pops up that needs dealing with. I received a call from the nurse at my doctor's medical centre. During the floods they were without power for thirty hours and since the vaccine for my desensitization is kept in their fridge, it now seems that it's been destroyed. Yep. I was asked by the nurse to ring my allergist to see if I could still use this vaccine. I did and was told it was very resilient, that it could even be frozen and thawed and that it was still ok, as long as it was not exposed to direct sunlight. I rang the nurse back and told her all this. Yay, all is good... or is it?

Off I went to my appointment with my doctor. I nearly didn't go, I am so tired sometimes, but I pushed myself, it's too important not to go. I have learnt to give myself a few extra hours to get ready if I have to go out, so yeah, getting a bit of a routine going, it may be the routine of a 100 year old, but it's still a routine.

I rocked up for my appointment and was met by the nurse with a hug saying, "Jenni you have to talk to your doctor in regard to your vaccine." All I could say was, "What? What has changed in two days?" Two big wigs higher up in the food chain than my allergist are giving out conflicting information about the safety of my vaccine. One is saying it's ok, the other is saying it is not ok and needs to be destroyed. I am saying bloody feckin fabulous!

Wow! Ok! Is this a joke? Am I being "punked"? Where are the cameras? Am I on a TV show that keeps putting obstacles in my way to see how long it takes for me to crack? Hmmm? Well? Geez! I feel like laughing, but I'm afraid it's of the hysterical kind. My doctor and I agreed that it wasn't safe to have my needle. I am not putting that in my body now regardless of how natural it is. You wouldn't eat an orange that had fur and penicillin growing out of its pith onto its peel, so yeahnah, "pith off", not having the needle now.

We have to wait for calls to be made to get new batches made up. Not only do I have to wait a few more weeks for my needle, I may have to pay another $195 to get the batch. If I blow up like a blowfish in the mean time, I will take a photo of it and put it in the book. A bit of light entertainment is needed at times I say!

The good news is we had a chat about the natural progesterone cream. My doctor looked it up and found it. I can get it on a script, but it isn't on the PBS list. I am going to have to try and change that! Time ran out, so back to him next week. The natural progesterone cream is made up with different percentages of ingredients depending on your need so we are working that out next visit. How? No idea, but will let you know. You didn't think it was going to be just straightforward and uncomplicated, did you?

I did go and chat to the local pharmacist. He explained that he couldn't mix it there as I have to go to a - wait for it - Specialist Compounding Pharmacy. Hey! Wait just a bloody minute! Is it in the deep jungle of a country I can't pronounce, where I will be swinging from vine to vine with a knife held in my mouth with the beating of drums in the background? Is it? No it's not? It's not far from home? And you have the number? Ok mate! What's the punch line? There is no punch line? Really? Wow, thank you. Phew! We all know I would have slid down the first vine and ended up stabbing myself in my eyeball or in my anatomy somewhere when I crashed hard to the ground!

Next I spoke to the Pharmacist at the Compounding Pharmacy. Originally I was told they don't "do" this cream. When I questioned her on why then is it available on script here in Australia, she went and checked with one of the "Compounders." Back on the phone there was a sorry with a comment about learning something new, but the best part was when she said yes they do "do" this natural progesterone cream with the yam origin. Bingo! The pharmacist explained that there is synthetic progesterone, the one I used with the HRT, it still makes me shiver and gives me nightmares! There is also BHRT, Bio-Identical Hormone Replacement Therapy. This, the pharmacist explained, is apparently close to the same hormones, as it is produced naturally in your body. And there again our knowledge bag about BHRT gets

129

fuller! Celebration! I know I am most probably celebrating too soon, but I like this feeling, so I am going to run, well, I am going to slowly walk and shuffle - with it. NB, old peoples shuffling not the shuffling done at clubs. The difference? My feet don't leave the floor!

Learning now that there is synthetic HRT, Bio-Identical hormones and foods that have natural estrogen and progesterone in them, I didn't even think to ask what was in the HRT that I used, well suffered through. How's that? I walked blindly into something with just faith in the medical community to keep me safe even though I originally wasn't going to touch it with a ten-foot pole! Haha, hehe, chuckle chuckle, how silly was I?

I still don't know exactly what is in them, but the words "animal hormones" has been a comment I heard just recently. I don't know, but HRT to me is becoming like the "snag" one throws on a bar-b-que. You never really know what is in it, but what you do bloody know is, it's going to have animal body parts in it that you would not normally ask for at the butcher.

What I do know from my research is that pregnant mare's urine is used in some HRT, but after learning *how* they collect the urine, I have made the decision that no other female, whether human or animal is suffering for me again. Have a look at PETA's website. The way these horses are treated is shameful, and as for their foals, well, they either take the place of their worn out mums or are slaughtered for the European food market. These majestic animals are made to suffer for us, for a product that will more than likely kill us in the long run.

Pharmaceutical companies who patent these HRT products don't care. It is and always has been about the dollar. Am I any better though? No I am not, even though I have never eaten horse, only attempted to ride one. I am not a vegetarian, I need to look at my eating habits and make some changes. I am so glad I am going to give the natural yam origin progesterone cream a go. I really hope it works for me, because as far as I know, yams don't have feelings!

Chapter 21

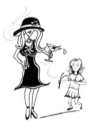

DEAR PRIME MINISTER

The pharmacist also gave me the phone number of The Pharmaceutical Benefits Scheme (PBS). I rang them to find out how I start trying to get this on the PBS. I was advised I had to ring the Local Member of Government with a letter as to why it should be on the PBS and he sends it off to the PBS in Canberra.

Ok, I just met the local Councillor the other week when he came around after the floods and we had a chat. Nice young bloke, hopefully he remembers me. At least it is a contact.

I found out through this Councillor's office that I need to do this through my local Federal Member of Parliament. I have all the details I need, I just have to organize a meeting and prepare my letter and myself to actually do this! I know I can send the letter to his office, but I would like to do it face to face, however I don't know if I have it in me. I wonder if he can come to my lounge room instead. I suspect not!

In my life prior to Ms Menopause I would have been "in like Flynn," what a great cause to fight for. Now, I am already feeling a bit jittery and stressed just thinking about it. I will just have to fight through this though, it is just so important to try and get this on the PBS list.

I know all this talk about getting Bio-Identical Hormones on the PBS seems very premature considering I haven't tried it yet, but from what I have learnt so far on this journey, nothing is just cut and dry when it comes to anything with Ms Menopause or the menopausal woman. I want to make sure I have all in hand, ready to go when needed.

I really did not feel too comfortable having to send this through my local Federal Member. It is nothing to do with going out of the house or preparing for it, I just want to make sure it gets into the right hands. Whose hands are those? No idea. So I have decided to go straight to the top. I have decided to send the request to our Prime Minister. There may be some of you who were reading this book with a nice cuppa, who just nearly choked on it. I could imagine, perhaps, some of you just sprayed coffee everywhere. I have looked into it and yes, we can send either a letter or an email to our Prime Minister.

To clarify, it has been sent to our first female Prime Minister. I felt this needed to be mentioned as I am hearing there may be a mutiny coming against her in the not too distant future and who knows who will be running the shop by the time this book gets published! I just hope it's not that bloke who is trying to turn this country back into the 1950s.

From what I have learnt, HRT is killing women with its many side effects because it causes more estrogen dominance. Menopause itself is killing women with the loss of hormones that do affect our health in so many ways. We lose all our progesterone and keep some estrogen, but at a lower level. Even without any therapy we will suffer with estrogen dominance naturally.

I didn't have this knowledge when I began with this whole bloody thing, but I do know I have to put hormones I have lost back into my body if I want my quality of life back, and I know I will not touch HRT again. Why they are still allowing it to be sold is beyond me, when we know now we get estrogen dominance naturally. Add HRT to the mix and it's like a double dose of estrogen dominance.

Now it all makes sense and is logical that I suffered so much more with bloating etc while I was on HRT. I also want something that is safe, natural and won't give me a period again - like I want to have to deal with all that for the rest of my natural life! I still suffer terribly with bloating, but it seemed to be twice as bad on HRT.

I need to really try to get it on the PBS list so every woman, regardless of finances, has the option to use it if she wants to. The cost I was quoted for 2013 were $63 to $85, depending on whether you need one percent or ten percent of progesterone. I will clarify for you how they determine the percentage for your personal needs, and how long a $63 amount will last you as soon as I know.

I also rang Paul back. He was the first pharmacist I spoke to who put me onto the Compounding Pharmacy. I wanted to know what the cost of this would be if it were on the PBS list. I was advised the cost is $36 if a woman does not have a health care card, and if one does have a health care card the cost is $5.90. Gigantic difference. Considering, well I assume, that it will be a lifetime need, this gives every woman a chance to use it if they choose to.

This is the email I sent to our, then - not the middle one and not the current one - Prime Minister:

Dear Prime Minister,

As an Australian woman who has been dealing with Menopause since 2010, I am requesting that you consider, please, putting Bio-Identical Hormones on the PBS list. It is available on prescription from doctors but the cost would be out of many women's reach at $60 to $80. On the PBS list the cost to a woman would be $36 or if a woman holds a health care card, it would cost $5.90 at 2013.

HRT and the side effects that come with it are killing women. Menopause itself, without any therapy is killing women. Women are living in old age with diseases, illnesses or conditions that are being put down to old age, but even though many of these are blamed on old age, they purely stem back to menopause.

Menopause is the peak time when woman are attempting or are actually committing suicide due to menopause-induced depression, but even this is being dismissed by the medical community.

These Bio-Identical Hormones allows a woman a safer option, if they choose, instead of having to use the dangerous HRT to try and alleviate their suffering. All women of Australia and the world will go through menopause and have to deal with its symptoms regardless of their walks of life or whether they have children or not. Seventy-five to eighty percent of women suffer through it and many find the journey debilitating.

In my dealings with it, I also have realised there is nowhere in society, or any of the government departments, that assists menopausal women. Centrelink offers payments for all needs except menopausal women. I personally have lost my earning power. Our workplaces cater for all forms of leave, except for menopausal women. I had to walk from my job where I was happy. As for our health system, in many cases, a woman's suffering through menopause is not listened to or taken seriously. The facts and truth of how menopause really affects a woman are also being surrounded by much secrecy.

Education and the truth, if given to women earlier, will allow a woman to be in control of her own health and retain her life and herself. It will also have a more positive ripple effect in our society if women are able to go into the last chapters of their lives healthy, happy and able. More importantly, loved ones will be a lot happier to see the older women in their family unit healthy.

Menopause needs to be put in the spotlight. There is no real menopause awareness, respect or support for menopausal women. I have also found that needs in menopause are not cheap. That includes medications, appointments tests etc. The average age is fifty-one, but women nowadays are going through it in their thirties, forties, fifties and sixties and are still dealing with it or an illness related to it in their seventies and eighties. Thank you for considering this request.

Well, that's done, hope I spoke ok on behalf of all woman who may be suffering. I also hope I get an answer, yay or nay.

Chapter 22

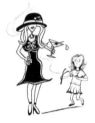

HEALTHY VS UNHEALTHY

Remembering that Ms Menopause is that one visitor who never leaves, what woman who is retired and living on the age pension could afford the $85 for BHRT? From what I hear, all pensioners have a hard enough time putting food on their tables. These women still play a very important part in their families' lives and in society, helping with grandchildren and sharing their many years of life experience and wisdom with the next generations. Allowing women to have quality of life at this time of their lives is not only their right, but will be of much greater benefit to women and society in general in terms of productivity and well-being. Now this is only looking at a woman who deals with menopause at the average age of fifty. Imagine the impact it would have on a woman who is dealing with menopause at an earlier age.

I think that Ms Menopause's arrival in my life in my mid-forties is fair. I don't think it is fair that in my early fifties I feel like a 100 year old. This could have been avoided with correct information and treatment. I really would not want to have to deal with this into my eighties. Yes I know that Ms Menopause will still be in my life then but I don't think I would be able to do the "hard yakka" in my eighties that I have had to do so far in this battle.

I feel for younger women who deal with this in their thirties and early forties as women will live with symptoms for the rest of their lives. I know firsthand that many people are subject to illnesses during their lives that are untreatable or unavoidable, but the issue I have is with the illnesses that rear their head due only to Ms Menopause. While only one percent of the population may deal with cancers, five percent with diabetes, ten percent with asthma and allergies, and fifteen percent with depression, one hundred percent of the female population will go through menopause.

Healthy older women: Have the choice to stay in the workplace after retirement age, still pay taxes and are productive. This then adds to the economy as we have earnings to spend. We are still paying into our superannuation funds for our retirement years. When we retire, funds for it will all still be there. For women who stay at home looking after families, their partners can go to work knowing that all is being looked after and cared for at home as they earn the dollars needed for their family unit. For all women, whether they are in the workplace or doing domestic duties, we are not a strain on our health system and Centrelink system, we are a healthy viable part of our family unit who are able to help with grandchildren, and are there for the emotional support of our family, partners, children and adult children and there to share our wisdom. We are there in mind body and soul, physically, emotionally and mentally, for the whole family unit and for ourselves.

Hell, we might not even be interested in any of the family stuff, a woman might prefer to get acquainted with her partner again after many years bringing up children or a woman might want to just actually find that partner. A woman might have big plans of travelling later in life, or plan to keep her successful moneymaking business running, or she may just want to sloth on her lounge, as she knows she has worked hard for this privilege. One might just want to be in the audience for the final of a Eurovision Song Competition one year (Smiley Face). The sky is the limit for women who, with knowledge, maintain health through menopause.

Don't assume we girls are now only good for the babysitting duties in our later chapters and also don't assume an older woman, if healthy, hasn't got money to spend. I have never been rich, well not in money terms, but with my health intact, I would still be out there gathering my dollars to run amok a bit more now.

Unhealthy older woman: Loss of earning power, not paying taxes or contributing to super funds. We will live on money that we should not have to touch until we retire from the workplace. We haven't the health to assist with helping with grandchildren, if we have them, and this then puts a strain on our adult children's family due to cost of child care. Adult children may have to take on care of an older woman, which not only affects their lives but will also lead to a strain on Centrelink. We become a strain on aged care facilities due to ill health with Alzheimer's disease and more. We also become a strain on our health system presenting with diabetes, osteoporosis, depression and cancer to mention a few. We are a strain on Centrelink as we are unable to work, so we may need to claim a payment before we are eligible for the age pension, and that in itself may not even be there in future years.

We lose our quality of life. Our relationships are severely affected and our loved ones miss and grieve for us, even though we are still here, but we are not who we used to be before going through "The Change." To be honest, I have grieved for myself at times. Regardless of whether a woman has worked in the workplace or worked in the home, the ripple effect of an unhealthy menopausal woman is huge.

Ok, that is my sliding door moment, what if I had walked into this phase of my life with education, knowledge and preparation? I'm sure there will be some out there who think this is all about retaining my youth. "She just can't accept the fact that she is getting old." I personally don't give a damn, but wanted to mention it because this is what we get thrown at us when we are searching for our health and wellbeing. I fully understand the concept of getting old, and the fact that our whole being is going to wear down with all those years of use, both mind and body. But to those who don't see or who choose not to see what is happening to women in menopause, that could be avoided. Well all I can say is, while I am still breathing I hate the thought of women suffering unnecessarily. I will fight for education and to make all the stupid, ignorant and flippant remarks made about Ms Menopause a thing of the past. Geez am I standing up for her again?

Many women I know who are in the workforce are doing their thing but are still struggling with improper care of their health in regard to Ms Menopause. If nothing else, BHRT will give a woman an option other than HRT. I know I will have a battle on my hands, as we all know HRT is a billion dollar business, but I think I am up for it, maybe, even if I have to do a bit of sobbing throughout my quest, have a nap in between it and carry that cushion for my gut to hang out on.

Chapter 23

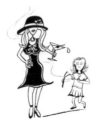

GOOD NEWS, CLARITY AND THE ARRIVAL OF "THE WHO FROM WHOVILLE"

An update on my desensitization needles. I received a call from the nurse saying that they have just received confirmation from France stating that my vaccine is still ok, even though they were without power for thirty hours during the floods. Yahoo! So I have my next needle on Monday instead of having to wait a few more weeks.

You know between my urine having to be sent down to New South Wales for testing, my cocktail mixture for my needles coming from France, and my natural progesterone cream having to be mixed at the Specialist Compounding chemist, I feel pretty special at the moment. Yeah! No backyard testing or mixing of ingredients for this "Meno Chick!" only the best will do. I will also be getting my script for the natural yam based progesterone cream, BHRT. Honestly I yam so excited!

Well I've had my needle and I have my natural progesterone script in hand. Off to the Specialist Compounding Chemist I go! We had to put a hold on getting the script though because it was all a bit confusing. No surprise there! I know now there is a saliva test that can be done to see how much progesterone is in my body, the cost to me is $50, and this will help determine the percentage of yam origin progesterone needed in my cream. I knew there had to be some way the progesterone level is worked out.

The original script given by my doctor, it was decided, started half way. The script my doctor can give me is either one percent, three and a half percent or five percent, so it was originally agreed we would start in the middle at three and a half percent. It's just all so full on, isn't it? I just want to sit in some corner and guzzle scotch and have a ciggie (oh no daughter, the ciggie part was only put in for dramatization!) and put my brain in a box for a moment, just like the good old days! So the results for the saliva test will take two days to come back, I then need to see my doctor to ensure the three and a half percent progesterone is right for me and if so I will get started on the cream. Oh I am just so bloody exhausted thinking about it all! I need to have a nap!

I need to add here how wonderful my doctor has been. I know he struggles with all this menopause stuff at times, but he has always been there for me. He has always listened and been respectful and taken the time to help me. If he finds out new information or snippets of news regarding Ms Menopause he always has it for me at my next appointment. I know he advised me to go on HRT after my visit to hospital but I know he was trying to do his best for me in the "box" he is allowed to practice in. I am starting to realise that maybe even doctors' hands are tied by to the powers above when it comes to the menopausal woman. So again to you my wonderful doctor, much gratitude, for all you have done and all you are still doing.

When I was talking to the pharmacist about this, I asked her what the rest of the cream was made up of since the yam base progesterone only made up three and a half percent of it. She told me it was macadamia based. Bloody hell, glad I asked! I know I get annoying as I don't stop asking questions, but geez almighty! With all the allergies I have it would have been a sure thing that I would have swollen and exploded if I started putting this bloody cream on my skin! Really? A nut based cream? Terrific! Really? I am getting a different cream base called "Versabase," cream that they can make easily, which is suitable for me with all of my allergies but bloody hell, thank God I asked!

We are now in the middle of February 2013 and it continues to be a challenging start to the year - are you starting to get bored yet? After having my needle and feeling pretty damn happy with a script for the natural progesterone, I woke up a few days later with swelling in my face and my top lip right up to the base of my nose was very swollen. I looked like a "Who from Whoville!" (Dr Seuss character). I wish I could have taken a photo of this, the "Who" look suits me!

I had to go to the doctor to get the form for the saliva test and the girls at reception suggested I get the nurse to have a look at the swelling. Of course when she saw me, I was sent into my doctor who had a look and checked my throat and lungs, then sent me back to the nurse where I had to get a steroid needle that had a general anaesthetic in it - to be jabbed in my bloody bum! Over it!

Yeah, this day was what I call a crying day. First the "Who from Whoville" look and all the discomfort and pain that comes with it, then the jab in my bum, then a comment that officially peeved me off. A bit confusing I know because I sound peeved all the time. Maybe I was just delicate because as soon as I spoke to a loved one I started crying. I have, though, I think, hit the nail on the head in regard to the medical world and society's attitude when it comes to the menopausal woman.

It is becoming quite clear that for a long time women have been intimidated into thinking that they haven't got the right to want to know more about Ms Menopause, and the attitude of "it's all a part of getting old" and "it's something we have to go through so just accept it," is still very much the accepted attitude around the world.

Yes I agree that menopause is a part of all women's lives and I fully accept it. I do not accept the attitude that dismisses a woman's suffering through it. Ms Menopause is not a natural part of old age. Drop that little clanger on a woman who has Ms Menopause knock on her door in her younger years. Yes I agree that my fifties mean I am middle aged, oh really, that went fast, but again, menopause is not a part of old age. It is a natural part of a woman's life. It is purely the ceasing of our monthly period cycles and the end of our childbearing days, nothing more, nothing less. If they say that fifty is the average age for women to start dealing with Ms Menopause, well fifty is my middle age, not my old age, so as usual, I beg to differ with their nonsense. Women are being intimidated and made to feel petty for wanting answers about their difficulties with Ms Menopause. This is a form of controlling women. Charming eh! Personally, I have never been backward in coming forward, so the more they try and squash me in relation to my right to find the answers I seek for myself, my daughter and any woman who needs help in this phase of their life, the more I'm gonna keep looking.

By doing this to women, it proves that they are hiding something, and this something is just how gigantic Ms Menopause is and how she can have such a debilitating effect on women. Well, you know what? They picked the wrong menopausal woman to try and intimidate, push around, and relegate my suffering to just old age. Yeah, "I am woman, hear me roar!" I am also very tired! Yaaawn.

Another thing I realised is that in the 1800s and even up to the mid 1900s a woman was considered old in her fifties. So this attitude we menopausal women have to deal with in the 21st century is still very much alive in the medical community and society itself. This is lame! They can make all sorts of advancements in other fields, but nobody gives a stuff about the menopausal woman. Yeah, there will be some who go on about the virtues of HRT, but we all know they would not have done that if it wasn't going to be a billion dollar business despite it's dangerous side effects.

I may be struggling to regain my health, my life, my whole being, hey I don't even know if I will get my health back, but I do know that the more resistance shown towards me, the more this chook becomes resistant to the attempts that try to stop women finding the truth and the attempts to disregard a woman's voice and the obvious need for safe therapies, support and respect while navigating their way through menopause.

Now, to the comment that peeved me off. Whilst sitting in the nurses' station waiting to have a needle in my bum - it just makes it all so much more serious when you have to have it in your bum, even when you are sitting there looking like a "Who" - the nurse who had previously stated that "'we' don't think it is a good idea to bombard women with all that can happen in menopause" was there for whatever reason.

We said hello to each other and she asked me what I had done to myself. I explained it quickly and we had a bit of a chat and yes, guilty, I had a bit of a bitch about Ms Menopause. Her next comment was, "Oh well it's all a part of getting old." Now to remind you, I am sitting there like a "Who from Whoville", my face is swollen a bit and I am feeling like death warmed up. I then said, "I haven't got a problem with getting old, but I do have a problem with everything that menopause is "pegging" at me.

Geez almighty! Ok then just to let you know, we all turn into "Whos" in old age, ok? Got it? Everyone comfortable with that? Bloody hell! I couldn't believe the comment. That is twice that woman has made those comments, a woman, go figure! I am a great believer that everyone deserves three chances, so this woman has one left. It may have to get to the stage where I have a quiet chat to her behind closed doors about her attitude and comments on menopausal women. In saying this though, and putting Ms Menopause to the side for a moment, this nurse is a really lovely person and has always been terrific with me in regard to taking blood etc, but…! It's just mind blowing to me, but not surprising, that another woman, who has spoken to me a little about her own experience with Ms Menopause, is telling women it is just old age.

She has the right to deal with Ms Menopause in exactly the way she feels is right and comfortable for her, but she does not have the right to turn the suffering of other women into something trivial by putting it put down to old age. I had a needle in my bum people. Whilst I was bent over waiting for it not one trivial thought entered my mind. This woman thinks it is funny when we have memory loss. I can tell you now it will not be funny if the day comes when your loved ones are heartbroken because you don't recognise them anymore. I know it sounds harsh, but for many women this will be the outcome of their journey with Ms Menopause if more isn't done to bring it out into the open. I pray to God I will not be one of those women.

I too have had moments. I took the remote for the TV to work in my handbag, I realised this when looking for my car keys to go home. I placed the candles in a birthday cake upside down, I realised when a mate of the daughter brought it to my attention, and no, I hadn't sneaked in a scotch! So, ok, I do get that in the beginning there may be a couple of funny moments, but later when you stop mid sentence because you cannot remember what you were saying or you forget what something is called or a thought you had just seconds ago disappears, and you try so hard to remember what that thought was, well it starts to get scary.

The "Who from Whoville" look is gone now, it took a few days. You know I kind of miss it. Putting the swelling, pain and discomfort to the side, there was, in a really strange way, something very comforting in looking like a "Who from Whoville." It conjures up hugs, kindness and all things warm and fuzzy. Maybe it's just me, I dunno.

Chapter 24

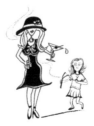

HAPPY ST VALENTINES DAY

So, did any of you have a lovely St Valentine's Day? What did I do I hear you ask? Well thanks for asking. When I arose from my slumber and glided out of my boudoir with my sexy bed hair, in my half torn off silk nightie after a very passionate night of romance, - you ain't believing this, are you? - on this very big commercialized money-grabbing day, I had to spit into the specimen jar for half an hour to collect my saliva for the progesterone test. Yep, all about romance here, lucky I am single!

Or maybe I should be saying lucky for that "gawjuz boy," that I used to stare at on many an occasion, that he had no interest in me whatsoever. Imagine if that had materialized! I would have ended it as I don't have the energy or health to deal with that even though I thought he was beautiful and he would have run for the hills when he realised my relationship with Ms Menopause was bigger than him and me. I'm saying it's a win-win situation. La la la. Moving on...

I didn't realize the spitting thing would take so long. Fair dinkum! You think you have heaps of saliva all for the taking, until you need to produce it. Oh and the arising from slumber? The reality was that after a night of snoring my head off and waking up nearly every two hours, I woke up puffy and groggy feeling like crap and even better, looking like crap. I stumbled out of bed in the t-shirt and shorts I found in the washing basket, I did the spitting thing, ensuring, as I am still half asleep, that I am actually spitting into the jar and not on the dog; yes she is still with us at the tender age of fifteen, I believe that is roughly 105 in doggy years.

I then groggily stumbled to the kitchen to eat so I can take the medication I need daily just to function. As for my hair, if it's still not in the ponytail, I am looking like a wild haired woman from the Stone Age, except I am cleaner as we have showers today.

I swear blind if I was a bloke I would have be giving my scrotum a good scratch on the way to the kitchen too bro. Yes, a very attractive St Valentine's Day look indeed. No "Fifty Shades Of Grey" here kiddies, just "Fifty Shady Symptoms" of Ms Menopause!

Oi! Ms Menopause, have I told you lately that I really don't like you? Oh, I have? Good, and what's with your name? Men-o-pause? It's even got the word men in it. What is that? Me is starting to thinketh you have your own cabaret drag show on the side.

I am sorry that I have to talk about my spit readers but it's all for the good of your health to know it isn't a thirty second job, because that's how long I originally thought it would take. A tip: if you need to collect your spit rub under your chin. That's what I was told and it works to produce more saliva faster. Off it went for testing, and back it came in the two days I was told it would take, see, miracles do indeed happen!

My results came back showing that I have a progesterone count of less than one. When the nurse rang with these results her words were that my progesterone level was abnormal, but I don't agree. Huh? I hear you say. My results are not abnormal, my result of a near to nothing progesterone level in my body is very normal and in line with how a woman's hormones are affected by menopause.

147

Getting the saliva results made me realise that I have learnt a lot and have got so much more knowledge on menopause, and my results prove that yes, I do know what I am writing about. Wow, I did know that, but now I have the physical proof of my results to prove it.

It also made me sad and a bit scared, but all my results do. Writing about it is very personal, but still a little impersonal in a way, compared to physically getting them. I admit my mind does shut down for a bit when I get my results; at times it gets too big for me to fathom and I usually go into denial or a "will think about how enormous that is later" sleep. This sleep is different to the wee amount of sleep we get with insomnia. It is different to the menopause-induced depression sleep, and is nothing like the "crap I just ate something that I should not have" sleep. It's more of a wave of sleepiness that comes over me, maybe it's just my mind going into overload with the results of the tests, and it needs a break from it all for a short time.

I guess it's the time when mentally, I take my big girl boots off. I go to the middle of nowhere in this sleep, so I don't have to think about it all for a moment. It's as if my subconscious mind has taken over and can digest and sort the bigness of it all for me as I sleep. Well that was pretty damn deep and profound. This "invisible" menopausal woman who has "no purpose" will give Sicko Fraud a run for his money any day.

My journey has begun with BHRT the natural yam origin progesterone cream. Yes I got it compounded and came home with my very own container full of it and a syringe to measure the amount needed. It is still very much trial and error as to how much I need and how often, and I imagine it's going to need fine tuning, but considering I have a progesterone count of less than one in my body, something is better than nothing. By the end of this book I will be able to let you know the results.

Chapter 25

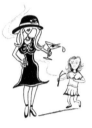

A QUICK BREATHER

So, onwards we go, and here we start the next twelve months of my journey with Ms Menopause. I am now fifty-two and it is 2013. *My fifties now officially suck!*

A bit surprised by the "now" bit? Yeah I know since Ms Menopause plonked herself down on my lounge back in 2010 it has all sucked! The battle to regain my health and feel like me again continues, but stuff happens and it just makes it all worse and all official!

Chapter 26

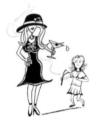

A VERY SAD DAY

I received an sms from the daughter at 4pm Aussie time on the 22nd of April 2013 to tell me Chrissy Amphlett had passed away. For those who don't know, I was a big fan of Chrissy's and her band The Divinyls. I turned the TV on and yes, sadly, there it was, Chrissy Amphlett had indeed passed away. Hearing the news just made me sob! The daughter rang me knowing I was a big fan but I couldn't even talk to her on the phone I was so upset.

The wonderfully wild, divine and talented Chrissy was only fifty-three. This fabulous rock chick passed away from breast cancer and multiple sclerosis. Well Chrissy, in my life and in my memory, of you I say: Thank you for paving the way for other rock chicks. Thank you for being the best female voice, in my opinion, to have ever come out of Australia. Thank you for being such a big part of my twenties and still a big part of my music that I continue to play in my fifties. Thank you for the music and for being you. You will be missed.

I saw the Divinyls in Tasmania in my early twenties with two mates. We were so close to the stage it was fabulous. The music and atmosphere was euphoric. Chrissy I was so happy to hear the rumours that you were all getting back together to go on tour. I couldn't wait to be in your audience again even if I was in my fifties, but this time I wasn't placing myself in the mosh pit, I was going to sit this time around! Well maybe. Oh ok, one foot in the mosh pit and one cheek on the chair.

Tonight the news said that we may see comets in the sky from 9pm until 4:30am. I say they are the universe's fireworks celebrating your life, or is it that you are already creating fireworks in heaven? In your own words I say "Hooroo." In my life, however long that is, you will never be forgotten. Oh and Ms Menopause is getting a bit snaky as I haven't written much about her yet. Bad luck daarling, I will get back to you soon. After all this time, have Ms Menopause and I come to a place of acceptance of each other? Well, no. She is still in control of my health, my life, actually everything to do with me. The only thing that has changed is that she has been able to do what she set out to do, and that is to take a back seat and make it appear that what I am going through has nothing to do with her at all.

The "M" word - MAMMOGRAM:

I decided I was going to have a mammogram in honour of Chrissy. Now. Breast screening, mammogram, hmm. I was supposed to have had mine a few years ago. At my age it's free, yes there are some positives to being middle aged, but as important as it is I kept delaying it. Stupid I know but the whole thought of it, what I have heard about it and what I have seen on TV, was very off-putting. I knew it was something that had to happen but I wasn't looking forward to it.

What I thought I knew about mammograms was that they squash your boobs down to the thickness of a frisbee, you had some stranger handling your "girls," and that it hurt. The day of the mammogram came. I really felt like a lamb being led to the slaughter and all morning I was not wanting to do it, but at the same time I wanted to do it in honour of Chrissy. Having to still deal with Ms Menopause wasn't helping either. So I arrived for my appointment and in time I heard, "Jennifer Townsend, when you are ready please come in." Chilling. I looked at the woman in front of me as she told me she was doing my mammogram today and I said, "Are you the same woman who was at reception?" Indeed she was, it was a bit creepy, a bit like "now you see me, now you don't," like, "Now I am a receptionist, now I am a breast screener." I was half expecting nipple clamps to appear. Geez.

Honestly, it was easy peasy! The woman did it very professionally and there wasn't a moment of awkwardness. She took four x-rays of my girls, they were not squashed down to the thickness of a frisbee, and it didn't hurt. And to let you all know, because we have no bone in our breasts, less radiation is needed - yes I found this out as I kept asking questions beforehand to delay it for another five minutes!

It didn't even feel uncomfortable having her position my boobs either. It was like she was playing with putty. "Yes Ms Breast Screener, feel free to mould my two girls into pert twenty-one year old supple breasts. As for the excess, yeah, just chuck it." Ladies, ensure you all have your mammograms. Honestly, it is not as bad as you may have heard and it is so important. Results here in my part of the world take ten days. If there are any problems they send you off to get it all double-checked. God willing, my two girls are healthy and okay but as always, I'll let you know.

Chapter 27

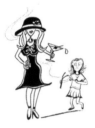

ANOTHER LETTER
AND JEAN HAILES

My March needle was done with nothing to talk about, yay! I still live on steroids daily just to function. I still struggle with Ms Menopause daily. Am I getting better? Well no. I have tried to go down 1mg of the steroids but within a day or two feel it and see it in my skin and within me. I also still have the bloating and I still can't deal with stress. It is also time to start looking for a new allergist but I will go into that later. I should be feeling a lot better than I am, shouldn't I?

Exciting news! I received a response to the letter I'd written to the Government asking them to put the natural progesterone cream on the PBS list. As we all know this is a part of the BHRT. I was impressed that I received the response in just under a month so thank you to the Australian Government which was running the shop at the time, before 2013. This was when we had our first female Prime Minister, so just ensuring that no one else gets or takes the credit when it isn't theirs to take.

It seems that it is up to the manufacturers of the ingredients that make up the BHRT - natural yam based progesterone cream - to submit a request to list this on the PBS. Ok then, now I need to get the manufacturer's information and shoot an email off to them. Oh hang on, I already have that information. Damn I'm good. Yes! I had a chat to a pharmacist soon after receiving this letter and was given the details I needed to contact the manufacturer.

I also asked her if she knew whether any natural products were already on the PBS. Her response was yes, there are two natural estrogens on the PBS already but they are manufactured by a different company. Ok then, I thought, can one woman make a difference? Let's wait and see. I sent off the email:

> Good Morning
>
> I am a fifty-two year old Australian woman who has, knowingly, been dealing with menopause since 2010. I have come to realize that the only real option that is being tossed at the menopausal woman in mainstream society is HRT. Many women, myself included, have turned their backs on HRT due to the dangerous side effects and illnesses it can create in a menopausal woman.
>
> HRT cannot be tailor-made to suit a woman's individual needs as it is mass-produced and tossed on a shelf purely for profit. After much research on my part I investigated BHRT and intend to trial the natural yam based progesterone cream.
>
> I am writing to you in the hope that you would consider putting a submission to list the natural yam based progesterone cream on the PBS list to the PBAC. This then would give every woman another option away from HRT and also bring the cost to a place that all women, regardless of their financial status, are able to afford if they choose to use it. I have also been advised that there are already two natural estrogens on the PBS list which are manufactured by a different company but unfortunately there is no natural progesterone on the PBS list.

Thank you for taking the time to consider this request and I look forward to your response.

So that's that! I had to let them know I was in Aussie-land because I am not too sure whether the email goes to Sydney or to the mother ship in America. Hopefully it will be a positive response, fingers crossed!

Going back to the response from the government and the fact sheet on The Jean Hailes Foundation that was enclosed, I thought I would look into this a bit more. Now Jean Hailes was a pioneer of midlife menopause and in 1971 set up the first women's health clinic dedicated to it. It is said that when Jean was going through her own menopause she researched it and, as a doctor, lectured on it. Jean was passionate about helping women in this phase of their lives and wrote a book in 1980 about midlife and menopause and from that book four actions were recommended on the *Jean Hailes for Women's Health* site:

- Know the facts: how menopause affects your body and emotions and what can be done.
- Keep yourself fit: to have a happy and productive life.
- Find a good doctor: if the doctor's attitude does not suit you, find one that does.
- Ask for a second opinion: it's your body and your life.

Jean Hailes, who was said to have made menopause respectable, passed away from cancer in 1988 at the age of sixty-two. The Jean Hailes Foundation was founded in 1992 in honour of all that Jean did. Then in 2012 her name was added to the Victorian Honour Roll of Women in recognition of her contribution to women's health. Wow! Thank you Jean for all that you have done.

I wanted to research the *Jean Hailes for Women's Health* site as this was all created four years after Jean passed away. I have to say I am a little disappointed that I still had to go searching for all my options. This is how my search went:

Typed in "Jean Hailes for Women's Health", ok I'm in. I find a wealth of information for all women even a statement that says, "Every woman has the right to a healthier life." Definitely agree with that statement. To the right, "Our websites", oh and there it is "Managing Menopause." It starts with "HRT - What you need to know." Ok I now speak out of ignorance as I did not read it all, but the little I did read was saying that HRT is now safe. So what has changed? Did the pharmaceutical company, due to the danger to women, change the ingredients? I don't think so! They say it is now safe for menopausal women of a certain age to use for a certain time. How do you know this? Where is your data that shows the facts on this now "safe" HRT? By data I mean where are the women who have used HRT and come out of it safely? I know what has changed. In Australia HRT usage has dropped by fifty percent, so what has changed is that billion dollar businesses' profit margins have dropped.

They also state there are different HRTs that need to be individualized, but this is blatantly false as HRT cannot be tailor made to a woman's individual needs. Oh, I see what you have done, you have made it *sound* like HRT can be individualized to a woman's needs but what you mean is that a woman has a choice of HRT in tablet, gel or patch form, so that is your very clever way of wording it to sound as if HRT can be made to a woman's individual needs. Readers, you read it and make up your own mind. As for me I am not touching it again with a ten-foot pole.

I can't see anything on our other option, BHRT, or any other natural therapies, so in I dig deeper and I type in 'natural therapies' but there is no way to enter my search, so I head over to the left side and search under 'Health A-Z'. OK I am at the 'Natural Therapies and Complementary Medicine' page. I am now scrolling right down this page that does have a lot of information but still there is not one mention of BHRT. Right at the bottom of this page under the *Jean Hailes* web pages is 'Complementary therapies used to treat menopause symptoms.' Click.

OK, again they talk about their views on complementary therapies, oh and there it is finally, 'Bioidentical Hormones.'

So, four pages in and quite a bit of search time before I finally found it – BHRT, buried under the front page which only talks about HRT and their views on it. I personally don't know how happy Jean would have been to know we still have to search for all our options on managing menopause. I know if it were me and a foundation had my name on it, I would want all the options to be on the front page. Who has time to dig that deep into a site? If you didn't know what you were looking for, you wouldn't find it here. Why, once again, is HRT the only option put out there as clear as day, and other options buried away?

OK, back to the 'Bioidentical Hormones' page. The first paragraph of the introduction says, "Women and health professionals are constantly being given information about "hormone imbalance" and how to deal with menopause "naturally". Really? You dare sit there and tell me that women are constantly being given information on how to deal with menopause naturally when you have buried all the natural therapies options, or what you call complimentary therapies. You dare sit there and again tell me that health professionals are constantly being given information on how to help a woman through menopause naturally when not once have I been advised by any professional of natural options except for some bloody useless herbal tablets. And finally, you dare to sit there and tell me these things when the facts and education are not out there to let women even know how big menopause is?

There is more in the introduction about how BHRT can be taken, but they forgot to mention that I very easily rub my cream into my arms and other places advised by my doctor, no need to suck my cheeks in! They also go on to say that there are false statements as to how natural BHRT really is. Try and make the time to read it yourself and again make up your own mind.

It then went on to talk about compound preparations which I feel came across in a quite unprofessional way. It stated:

Compounded "bioidentical" hormone preparations also require a doctor's prescription and are made up by the pharmacists who call themselves: Compounding Pharmacists. There are no further training requirements for compounding pharmacists, who are likely to have had the same training as your family pharmacist.

Well ouch! Very unprofessional people, and on behalf of all those wonderful, helpful and knowledgeable family pharmacists, how dare you? Who do you think you are once again trying to discredit not only BHRT but also pharmacists?

Oi and leave my compounder mates alone! What they have compounded, and I will say very professionally for me so far, has been exceptional, so pull your heads in. I don't think for a moment that if Jean were in control of her foundation, she would ever have allowed you to make such a distasteful and unprofessional statement, or to dismiss someone else's training for your gain. Yeah, your gain!

There is a lot more written about how bad BHRT is and how there are false and misleading claims in regard to the safety of BHRT, so again I suggest you read it yourself. Interestingly though, all their "Further Developments" on the evils of BHRT was in January 2008. I am sitting here now not even two months away from January 2014. So their "Further Developments" paragraph at the end is six years old? Hmm, I am using my BHRT and feeling better for it. So where is the up-to-date information on the evils of BHRT?

Jean, before I go on with this I want to say to you that you were a pioneer for the menopausal woman and I say it with much gratitude, thank you. I know this foundation was created in your name after you had passed away, I just wish you were still sitting at the helm, as after reading about you I know for a fact you would never have sold out womens' health for the almighty dollar. I know there is a wealth of information for women of all ages and at all stages of their lives on this website, but speaking as a menopausal woman it concerns me that your name is being used to sell HRT when there are other options.

A part of the fact sheet received from the Australian government also states:

> The Australian Government provides funding to the Jean Hailes Foundation to influence and resource women and health care professionals to achieve changes in attitudes and culture that encourage women to make informed choices about their own health care.

Firstly, I don't want to be "influenced," which I feel this foundation is doing, by people saying how good HRT is and how evil BHRT is, and having other natural therapies buried deep in the bowels of their website. I agree that I want to make informed choices about my own health care, but that becomes a bit impossible when we are not given all of our options openly and when all our options are not presented on an equal footing with HRT. It also becomes quite impossible to make any kind of informed choice when the information is not transparent.

Before I move on I have one question to ask the Board of Directors of the Jean Hailes Foundation: If you are truly there for the menopausal woman's health and wellbeing, if you truly believe that every woman has the right to a healthier life and if you are not profiting personally or for funding for the foundation by selling HRT, why are all the options like BHRT, natural therapies and HRT, not put on the front page of your "Managing Menopause" so that every woman can see all her options transparently, and can then make an informed decision as to what is best for her?

I find as I go further down the bumpy road of my journey with Ms Menopause that she herself is a large money making machine. I also have seen on many occasions that the negative thinking of society in the 1800s is still very much alive in the 21st Century concerning the menopausal woman. I have no doubt that "they" will even try to smear me as I am speaking up for BHRT. You know what though? I couldn't give a rat's ass! Give it your best shot, because as I always said to my daughter, the truth is always the best armour you will have when you go into battle for the things you believe in. So bring it on kiddies!

Wow, it's amazing how once you start looking into Ms Menopause she can branch out and wrap around us and strangle the essence of who we once were out of us but I was a bit surprised and actually elated to find the following.

I thought before finishing with the *Jean Haile's for Womens' Health*, which was originally called *Jean Haile's Foundation* I would google "What did Jean Hailes think about BHRT?" I don't know if BHRT was around before Jean passed over but I thought I would try and find out what Jean herself thought about it, and not all those who bandy her name around for the good of HRT and the evil of BHRT.

I came across a site which was called the *Medical Observer* with a title of "BHRT promo" dated June 2010. They were up in arms as Samantha in the *Sex in The City 2* movie was menopausal and was promoting bioidentical hormone therapies. The Jean Hailes Foundation for Women's Health, of course, got into it and said that the movie portrayed midlife women in popular culture as "slaves to their hormones." I'm thinking, "Yeah! And your point is?" We *are* slaves to our hormones due to the lack of transparency.

The Jean Hailes Foundation went on to strongly recommend that we see a qualified health professional to ensure that we are receiving the latest in evidence-based health and care information. I agree. I just find it a bit curious that this foundation gave this advice in 2010 after no BHRT updates in "Further Developments" since 2008.

So those speaking on behalf of Jean are basically talking out of their backsides as they have not given women any updated information on BHRT for nearly six years; so they just know that BHRT is evil, is that it? Or does it go back to the same old same old, that HRT is a billion dollar business and anyone who wants to be a part of it can also make some nice fat dollars!

Later I talk about the natural foods that contain the hormones we lose and other information that may help you. I always knew that I needed to see a naturopath to ensure I was giving you the best info in this book, but our belts are so financially tight that I knew I couldn't use money to see a naturopath yet.

I was at my local chemist - yes the one where all the compounders live - and noticed they had a new service for customers. A naturopath was at the chemist on Fridays and it was a free service for customers. Bingo! Of course I booked myself in for the following Friday. I spoke to the naturopath about the best foods and so on. I then asked her about BHRT. This naturopath told me there was a doctor who specialized in BHRT a bit of a drive away but still not too far from home. Double bingo! I wrote down his details and walked away knowing, again, once I had the funds, I was going to meet this fellow for sure! This time I wanted to be guided by a doctor who actually specializes in BHRT instead of winging it like the first time.

Unfortunately the May needle I had was a doozy! I wasn't feeling too good before it, but when you are feeling like crap most of the time, it becomes your normal. I'd had a little tickle in my throat before I had the needle and the start of a very small cold sore just under my nose. Well I was as sick as all sick after it. The days to follow started with sneezing, then full-blown 'flu with vomiting that lasted two days. I slept most of the time for days. My family wanted to take me back to the doctor, but I was too sick. I knew when I was feeling better I would get back to him.

When back at my doctor's after this "OMG what was that?" and after he checked me over and made sure I hadn't vomited up a vital organ or another bit of me which I needed, we had a good chat. He told me that because my immune system is already fighting so hard against my allergies, I am now more susceptible of catching germs and infections than ever.

Fabulous! The hormonal system is interconnected with the immune system, so just be aware of this when Ms Menopause comes knockin' at your door. For me it is my allergies, but it can do so much more. I also asked him to refer me to another allergist as I thought it was time for a second opinion.

Most days I really don't know what is going on with me health-wise. I have so many allergies and at times I feel like my food allergies are getting bigger. There was a time when I could eat and drink pretty well anything I wanted. We used to have a joke within our family circle that we all had what we called The Townsend Iron Stomach. I come from a long line of people who were able to eat and drink whatever they wanted. I was very happy with this as I am a woman who always enjoyed food.

My food allergies only worsened a bit after giving birth to my daughter but more so now that Ms Menopause has knocked. I find this interesting and I will speak more about it later. I will let you know though, I miss, to name a few, scrambled eggs, peanuts, cashews, smoked oysters, glasses of chardy, prawns, potatoes and the list just goes on and on. Oh and Pavlova!

I must admit I am over the continuous and constant struggle for my survival. I had just got my first lot of BHRT to start, but I didn't get into a long-term routine with it as I have been so sick. Some days it is a struggle just to get up and feed myself so that I can take the medication I need to function. Some days I sleep. But when I am feeling a bit better and get me some more funds I intend to get back into the BHRT. So my first attempt was a bit hit and miss with BHRT, so I am not too concerned about starting over again with it.

I received the letter from BreastScreen QLD stating that the results of my mammogram had come back clear and that my two girls are ok. A few of us were in the lounge room discussing it and we were all relieved and full of joy that I didn't have to deal with any more than I already am. At the same time though the news had just come on telly saying that Angelina Jolie had just come through a double mastectomy and reconstruction. Wow! Talk about a bittersweet moment.

I just stood there thinking I was so happy for me and my family, as I could see the relief on their faces, but I felt so sad for this woman I had always admired. My thoughts go out to all those women who are dealing with this terrible disease. I threw a prayer up to the universe for all of you. To my mate who has battled this and is also now dealing with other health issues, I asked the universe to especially look after you.

Chapter 28

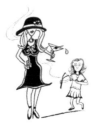

THE FIRST ALLERGIST

To summarize: In 1998 I discovered I was allergic to our new dog. In 1999 my doctor referred me to an allergist who did the skin prick test on me which showed I was also allergic to a few other things. I started on a year of desensitisation injections. In 2007 I worked with a chemical that affected me and the girl I worked with. Rashes, headaches and a cyst on my ovary appeared. My allergist did no testing and said I only had sinus. When I left that job all the symptoms disappeared. By the way, I have never suffered hay fever or sinus.

In 2010 Ms Menopause arrived and I started to get rashes again so I went back to the allergist. I should have asked to see a different one. In 2011 I had six months of fortnightly booster desensitization shots. My IGE (allergy rate) before these shots was 13,000. A normal allergy rate is zero to100. After these booster shots my IGE had risen to 16,000 by 2012. In mid-2012 I ended up in hospital and my IGE was now 22,300. I had to give up work due to these health problems and have not been able to work since.

I had asked my allergist once again if he thought menopause could be playing a part in all of this and he dismissed this idea. I continued on the monthly injections until July 2013 which I've now completed. He has, in my opinion, a lot to answer for, not only in terms of my health but also my finances. I began looking for a new allergist because I knew this middle-aged menopause woman was never seeing him again.

My IGE did go down minutely in January 2013, but it has since risen and is continuing to rise. My new allergist is booked and I see him early September 2013. My loved ones would look at me and say, "Are you sure the allergist got the right cocktail mix for you? He could be injecting anything into you." I would always come back with, "I just don't think he took Ms Menopause seriously enough." I will say though, I do have the vial of left over desensitization cocktail mix sitting in my fridge here at home if I ever feel the need to get it analysed.

The final needles in June and July were not too bad. The June one made me a bit dizzy and I had a bit of a cry in the waiting room. My daughter had come to support me. I think the May injection scared the "bejeebers" out of them and she insisted she come with me. Maybe they thought this time I might vomit up my posterior and turn myself inside out! I dunno! I was very relieved she was there for me because she held my hand as I sobbed. I love you my daughter.

Otherwise I am now done and dusted with the five months of booster shots and the yearly injections set up by the first allergist but I am no better. My skin tells me that; at times I would wake up and my face and eyes would be so swollen that I would have to push my puffy eyelid in so I could open my eyes properly. Geez maybe the loved ones were right about the wrong cocktail mix being made up for me. "See yar, don't want to be yar," first allergist. You and I will never meet again unless of course that cocktail mixture comes back with the wrong ingredients - if you get my drift! I don't think so though, as I was struggling with inflammation even before the injections started and even before needing steroids. Did the injections make my journey worse? Don't know. I still believe the first allergist just didn't take Ms Menopause seriously enough.

There have been, and continue to be, so many up and down events and so many up and down emotions since Ms Menopause knocked on my door. I guess though that is what life is about anyway, but the difference is that you get it all thrown at you once she turns up. So let's move on to a high note before we crash down to a low note.

OMG guess what! When my daughter and I were driving home from having one of my final needles, my daughter all of a sudden said, "Mum, do a u-turn, I just saw a big sign saying "Women's Health-MENOPAUSE." Of course we went and had a look. It was a big pink sign at the medical centre just a stone's throw away from home. We used to see our family doctor here but it had closed down and we lost contact with him for a little bit. We did find him again in 2008. This old centre had reopened a while back, but never had this big pink sign been on it before.

I went in as I knew I wanted to ask the question, "Do you have a doctor who deals with BHRT?" Yes they did, a doctor who thinks out of the box, they said, and his name is the same name I had been carrying around with me ever since the naturopath gave it to me. Wow! I now had this doctor who specialized in BHRT just down the road from home. It was exciting but it would have been more exciting if I had the funds to see him. But I knew the time would come when I would see this fellow. You know, when I got home and thought about it, why did I have to waste precious time to track down a doctor who "thinks out of the box?" Why aren't we given all our options at the beginning so that we can make decisions for ourselves earlier? Where are all the pamphlets on menopause Medical World?

Yeah it got me thinking, so the next time I was waiting to see my doctor I checked out all the pamphlets on display. I could nearly hear the other people thinking, "What is she trying to pinch?" Well Medical

Centre, if they were all in the same place instead of at each corner of the room I would not have had to do the "weirdo walk." Not one about menopause. Now this Medical Centre has lots of doctors and different services for patients, and there was not one pamphlet about menopause or even information to guide us somewhere. I know they can't cover everything, but we are not talking about a condition that only affects one person and which is baffling the medical world. Menopause affects every single woman, from every generation, right around the bloody world. I didn't tell my doctor about this "weirdo walk" but we did discuss getting me a new allergist.

As I walked in the next week for my next appointment with my doctor, I noticed there was a questionnaire on the receptionist's counter for us to fill out regarding the centre and its services. Well in my mind I went yes please, this will give me a chance to voice my concerns about there being no pamphlets on menopause in cooee of the medical centre. I filled everything out with 'excellent' until I came to the 'other' section. My first word in capital letters was POOR - the lowest choice - with my thoughts on it all, so we will wait and see if one woman *can* make a difference. I reckon it will go one of two ways: either it will make a difference, or the next time I try and walk through their sliding glass doors I will be warned off the premises. Who knows?

Throughout all of this, the last few monthly needles and the excitement of knowing the BHRT doctor was in walking distance from home, I knew that depression was lurking, as usual, and I could feel it raising it's ugly head again. This time though it came at me without warning. Sounds silly I know, but I had always thought I was in control of it and that it was a coward, as it would only show itself when I was alone.

Before I continue I need to remind you, actually no! I need to remind *me* of who I used to be before Ms Menopause. I was a strong independent woman with a strong body. I was always able to earn my dollars and care for my family. I did a little travelling before I settled down to do my most important job, that of being a mum. I had only ever been admitted to hospital once in my life and that was to give birth to the daughter twenty-one years ago. I had never had to depend on any form of medication in my life, but chose to hang with scotch and chardy on the weekend or Friday nights. Ciggies have been in and out of my life, but they were the only drugs I chose to put in my body. Oh yeah and I think I used to have a pretty damn good sense of humour.

I had to remind myself of all this. I don't know why but it just makes me think that maybe after all that I have gone through, perhaps the real "me" is waiting in the corner somewhere to come and take her rightful place again instead of this "me".

As I have said, I believe certain medications, if needed, do give back quality and happiness in peoples' lives. For me though, I want *my* normal back. I am finding it hard to fathom why the medical world feels that the way to fix a menopausal woman is always with steroids and anti-depressants.

Chapter 29

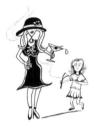

DEPRESSION AND
SUICIDE... AGAIN

And so depression raised its ugly head again. Most days I feel a bit sad, other days I feel the sadness surround and engulf me, but it feels different to the depression. I did feel a bit depressed in February but tried to push it aside as I was so excited about starting my BHRT. Well depression doesn't like being ignored and pushed to the side. I really am finding it hard to talk about, but again I need to, for all our sakes.

Depression came back with a vengeance and the way it came back quite shocked me. It grabbed me at a time when I tried to feel like me again for a moment. I actually thought that because I was aware of it I was in control of it, and it would normally try and grab me when I was alone, so I used to think it was a coward. I am tired of Ms Menopause controlling every aspect of my life and I get angry with her for the way she has been allowed to affect my family. I tried to "buck up" but found that it is quite impossible to do this without her digging a bigger hole for me. Actually Ms Menopause doesn't get her hands dirty, so it was one of her troops that dug that hole for me. This is what happened:

I am tired of all the bullshit I have had to deal with since 2010. I have fought a good fight against Ms Menopause. But I want to be me again! So one afternoon I decided I was going to be me again and I headed down to our local as I had decided to sit in the sun and enjoy a chardy as I had in the past. What I didn't know was that bloody depression had come along too.

Whilst sitting there sipping the chardonnay my thoughts just clicked over and I made a decision to commit suicide. I decided I was going to walk to where my sister used to live, then do it. Was this a conscious thought? No. For some reason it just felt like my thoughts had been taken over. I knew I was in there amongst it all somewhere, but I knew I wasn't in the driver's seat. To try and describe it, I felt like a robot being controlled by someone else. I finished the chardy and left my best mate an sms saying - well sobbing - that I couldn't continue to live like this blah blah blah, and then I started walking.

Fortunately the universe had other plans, and not long after I started walking I fell and hit my head, no other part of me had any scratches or bumps on it. It was as though I had been picked up from the back by both my legs and dumped down on my face. The left side of my forehead was cut and bleeding. And let me just say here, I have walked this path many a time before. Not once had I ever fallen over on it, even after a few chardys.

As I fell a few young people came to see if I was ok. Thank you for caring. It was at that time that I felt like "I" clicked back in and all I could say was, "I am a menopausal woman and I am scared that I am going to commit suicide." These beautiful young people stayed with me until the ambulance came and carted me off to the Mental Health Unit at a local hospital.

It is very hard to talk about this but it is too important not to. Why is it hard to talk about it? To be honest it felt like I was talking about someone else for a while, and also there is such a stigma in society that goes with it. I don't give a rat's ass what people think of me, I would think less of myself if I didn't talk about it, all of it, including the not so socially acceptable moments. Thank god I have never been the type to care what society thinks of me. I yam what I yam, and as usual I say, "If you don't like it, don't look!"

Menopause-induced depression is a very real thing, with or without a chardy. It needs to be taken more seriously and put in the spot light. Actually thinking about it, there are no socially acceptable moments with menopause in my experience. So Universe, you did choose the right girl to deal with all of this! Ms Menopause may have a strangle hold on my ovaries but you know I have always been a fighter for the under dog and that bullying is always a no-no in my books. I was never the type to just sit in a corner watching injustice being done without trying to do something about it.

I was involuntarily admitted to the mental health unit and I can tell you, the moment those doors close behind you and you find out that you are not free to come and go as you please is terrifying. I only settled down a bit when I found out they could only keep me for six hours. Yes I was happy to be there, I needed to be there, but nobody told me I couldn't go home when I wanted.

Actually it could have been a less terrifying moment if I had known and been prepared for those doors locking behind me and if I had known straight up that I could only be held for six hours. Hint hint, Mental Unit Ward! I did mention this to the team member while I was there and she said that yes they need to look into that. I am hinting at it here in case she forgot to "look into it."

I was there for three hours waiting and then being assessed by one of their team members. After talking it out, and after them ringing my loved ones to ensure our stories matched as to why I was like this, I was allowed to go home.

As I was walking out I said, "Don't fob off the menopausal woman." Interestingly there was another woman in there waiting to be assessed who heard a little of my talking. As I was leaving she said to me, "Your situation sounds familiar to me, but I am also in the process of losing my house." Yep this woman was my age.

I would have loved to be able to sit with her and chat, but I was too scared to sit my bum down in there again as I thought if I did, I get to stay another six hours and I just wanted to get home. I hope she is ok and being listened to.

I am sorry for my loved ones who have had to deal with this in all its enormity, but am also so proud of them as they have their own knowledge of the devastating effects Ms Menopause can have, and thus our stories matched. I am also very relieved that our stories *did* match. Geez the loved ones could have taken this opportunity to send me off on a long holiday, like *One Flew Over the Cuckoo's Nest*. I love you all. Thank you for not taking this opportunity to, you know, give us all a rest. I do feel at times that Ms Menopause is driving me crazy, but I don't think I was totally normal, whatever that might be, before she arrived. I used to pride myself on sitting on the edge and as I have always said, define normal. Yeah, I believe we all have our own normal and that is ok as long as it is not hurting anyone or ourselves. I just want to get back to *my* normal.

Oh and to let you know, there was not one bruise, cut, scratch, bump or sore bit on my body, only the damage to the left part of my forehead which is totally healed now. Initially I wanted to say, "A bit harsh don't you think Universe?" But now I realize it was the only way you could get my attention when I was in that state of mind. It really did knock me back to me, so now I say, "Thank you for loving me and stopping me from taking my life. I love you all." Suicide is not a legacy I want to leave to my loved ones and most importantly not to the daughter.

Chapter 30

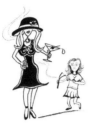

THE PSYCHIATRIST

After all this was said and done I had to see my own doctor who suggested it might be a good idea to see a psychiatrist. I am now a menopausal woman with a mental disorder due to losing those two main hormones. See how it seems to be moving more away from Ms Menopause? Psychiatrists specialize in the diagnosis and treatment of mental disorders. I didn't want to go but I felt I owed it to my loved ones, so off I went praying, "Please God, please don't let it be the psychiatrist from the Sunday paper that I bitched about earlier in this book." Thanks. Amen.

Well what can I say? He was a nice bloke, he asked me questions, he let me talk and then he decided I needed to be on anti-depressants even though he was unsure as to why I was dealing with depression. I did, of course, ask him if he thought that menopause had a hand in it. He said no. I also said that I realize that I may have played a hand in it by having a chardy. His response was that the chardy had nothing to do with it and he was sure it was going to happen anyway.

Ok. I understand that, but it concerns me that he wasn't concerned or didn't even try and give me a lecture on the dangers of alcohol and depression even if you are not menopausal and allergic to the stuff. Maybe it's not his job to do so. He did make a valid point though. He said that the brain is just an organ like any other organ in our bodies, so if it needs medication it is no different to say, the kidneys or the heart or whatever it is that requires medication. Cool eh!

I get that and if I need to go on antidepressants long term I will, but if there is another option for me as a menopausal woman I am going to try my hardest to find it before I alter "my" normal. "My" normal got me through life pretty damn well until Ms Menopause knocked. I imagine if any expert is reading this they would be thinking, "No it won't alter your normal, it will make you normal." Rightio, let's wait and see eh? Give me a look at that handbook "youse" carry around that defines normal. I've been looking for that book all my life.

All these experts make me question myself and at times I walk away from them thinking, "Am I barking up the wrong tree? Am I kicking a dead horse? Does Ms Menopause even exist? Who do I think I am, questioning the majority of these professionals?" But I know all that I am dealing with is Ms Menopause so why won't the Medical community give me a break and admit it?

I had to see my own doctor to discuss the psychiatrist's opinion in detail. I told my doctor I am not going to go on antidepressants. He was a little shocked, but he respects my decision, although he now wants to monitor me even more closely that he was before.

Oh and purely for the psychiatrist, I will now give you my expert opinion: I am a menopausal woman losing those hormones which affect us in so many ways. The name for my condition is menopause-induced depression. I hope that gives you a heads up in your next session, but I'm thinking you already knew that.

Whilst still with my doctor and feeling quite despondent about it all, I said to him, "There really is no expert on menopause is there?" He then said that I could go and see an endocrinoligist. They are doctors who specialize in hormones! Of course I said sign me up. So off I went praying that this hormone doctor had some miraculous healing powers or somefin'. And to all those dealing with depression, regardless of menopause or not, my heart goes out to you. I hope you are being treated with compassion and respect.

You know, before we meet the endocrinologist, a funny moment did happen on the way out of the psychiatrist's session. I say funny, many may say cringe worthy. Well, when my doctor organized this appointment he knew I was waiting on more pocket money to come so he set it up to cost me nothing. After the whole suicide thing he didn't want me having to wait. On the way out of my session I went to the receptionist counter to see if I had to sign anything. When the receptionist said that will be $70:

Me: My doctor told me there is no cost.

Her: Well your doctor had no right to tell you that!

(I was half expecting her to HISSS after she said it as she was getting a little snaky over this "ordeal")

Me: Well I don't know what you want me to do as I have no money on me!

Her: [Goes into his office, closes the door and no doubt, after mixing a martini and kicking her legs up on his desk, discusses this crisis!]

I had three thoughts as I was wandering around the waiting room looking at their pamphlets: I could do a runner but I haven't got the energy, how much washing up will I have to do to pay this off and just go home and ring through your card details. That's right, not even a credit card on me. I know what was in my purse at that time and it was a spare car key!

Her: [Comes out of doctor's room] It's OK, you don't have to pay.

I call her 'her' because I didn't like her even before she tried to swindle seventy bucks out of me. I didn't like the way she spoke to another guy that went in before me. Why is it that some people who deal with the public are such a.... holes? How hard is it to be respectful and polite? She was "Ginger Hard Nosed B..." for no reason and she needs to remember she is dealing with people who are a little bit more vulnerable. So she needs to pick her act up and show a bit more compassion towards others. Got it?

Look I know what working with the public can be like at times. At the job I thought I was going to retire from, I was the first to say I was glad my days of working with the public were over. But let's all remember, we all serve each other at times in life and we are all "the public" too. I was the front line person copping the abuse for the mistakes that were made by someone in the back bowels of the office. I even had a phone thrown at me once. He missed. I moved faster in my younger years.

Why did he throw it? Because this "pig" came into the financial institution I was working at and tried to withdraw money out of his wife's account without being a signatory on it. So this was always going to be a no regardless of his "pigness". He didn't throw the phone at me because I was rude; he was trying to intimidate me into saying yes to the withdrawal. So yeah, I get that working with the public at times can be pretty hard, but I still don't get 'her' attitude.

Maybe she was peeved as they had run out of olives to put in her martini or maybe the $70 I didn't cough up was to pay for more martinis. I am sorry to the shrink for the error, as for her ... Oh and just before we wrap this up they also had no information on menopause-induced depression. They had a large range of information on many other mental disorders including post natal depression, but nada on my menopause-induced depression, oh I mean, my mental disorder.

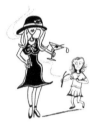

Chapter 31

THE ENDOCRINOLOGIST

What a lovely human being. This woman was really nice and very professional. We did the normal stuff, you know, getting my history blah blah blah, and had some great chats in between. This doctor could see the redness and rawness of my skin and I advised her I was seeing a new allergist in September, which was not very long after seeing her, and guess what? She knew him and told me he was one of the best in his field. "You beauty!" I thought. When she learnt that hot flushes and night sweats haven't been a biggie for me it was enough for her to decide not to suggest HRT for me. I would not have done it anyway.

I came away from that meeting with the endocrinologist suggesting the allergist might be my best bet, not in those words, but along those lines, so I was really no further down the track in regard to my health than I had been before seeing her. But a couple of really interesting facts came out of seeing her. Did you know that when you are pregnant your immune system is suppressed so that you don't reject the baby? Interesting eh!

Also I asked her why she felt that some women dealing with menopause suffered less with hot flushes and night sweats than others. Her response was that they thought originally women who were thinner had fewer hot flushes and night sweats. Well in my head I was thinking, "Take one look at me and that will throw that theory out the window. Not much thinness on this missy." But she then said that that has been proven to be incorrect.

I asked her if an endocrinologist is an expert on menopause. She said that if they wanted to specialize in menopause they could by doing further training. This hormone doctor hadn't. She also told me that she knows of endocrinologists who refuse to take on patients with diabetes. I don't know why, I don't remember asking her, but I always thought all these specialists chose these career fields to help people, not to pick and choose who they want to treat and to take astronomical fees from.

So to finish, thank you Endocrinologist, I really enjoyed talking to you. The fact about the immune system through pregnancy was really interesting. Thank you also for bulk billing me and getting me in a bit earlier when you learnt of my journey so far with Ms Menopause.

This now might be the right time to chat about pregnancy! What the…? Yeah pregnancy. As I travel down this long road with Ms Menopause I realize that menopause is just the other end of the spectrum. Before that knock on the door came, I never would have thought that these two were related at all. Call me a moron, but yes, I fell pregnant and gave birth to my daughter never really knowing what was happening to my body. Of course I knew I had to keep myself healthier and it took nine months and by now we all know that I definitely knew *how* to fall pregnant, but I also wilted throughout pregnancy. It got me thinking that I am wilting through menopause as well so there has to be a connection.

This is what I learnt. We have pregnancy and menopause, and we also have our monthly cycle beginning at puberty. Estrogen and progesterone are the two big players in these three life experiences of a woman. I also found the endocrinologist's comment that our immune system suppresses itself throughout pregnancy so that our bodies will not reject the baby interesting.

So as best as I can remember I am going to compare my pregnancy with my menopause.

MY PREGNANCY: I was elated and over the moon. I was thirty and I was ready. The smell of alcohol and vegetables cooking became vile to me. My skin needed more moisturising than normal. I had intended to work right up until a week or two before my baby was due, but because I was wilting I had to leave work earlier. I gave birth to my beautiful girl but had a few complications. Severe blood loss meant I nearly died and I had to be whisked away for surgery and have blood transfusions. I had to spend two weeks in hospital. I can't remember whether I had any cravings.

Once home I was having a bath whilst all the loved ones cared for and were still in awe of this beautiful little addition to our tribe. Whilst in that bath I had a very fleeting thought, "I could just put my head under the water and drown myself." I spoke to my sister about this and was advised that I was dealing with post-natal depression. My hormones re-aligned, I never had a thought like that before my pregnancy nor after that moment, well not until Ms Menopause turned up twenty years later. I had a year off work with my new daughter and on we went living our lives. The only two differences now were that my allergies came to the fore in a very small way and that I was a fully-fledged mum. How did I ever breathe before this little girl came into my life?

MY MENOPAUSE: I was elated and over the moon, party time! I am allergic to alcohol and pretty well most things. My skin, well we all know about that. I had intended to work right up to the age of seventy, but due to wilting and finding out that menopause actually sucks, which we all now know shouldn't be the case, I had to leave work earlier. I

179

have had nothing but complications with my menopause and at times I have honestly thought I was going to die. I have been admitted to hospital twice so far since my menopause started. I have bled to the extent of feeling like I am haemorrhaging, but this time it was caused by a man-made product called HRT.

I think I did have a craving. I was eating whipped cream a lot even to the extent of buying those aerosol cans of whipped cream and topping Jatz biscuits with it. I would also just tilt my head up with the whipped cream can in hand and spray it straight into my mouth! I have been dealing with menopause-induced depression. My hormones in this part of my life will not align. It is all loss, loss and more loss. I have not been able to work now for eighteen months and I am trying to get my health back to a place where I can go on living my life. The main differences now are that I have a bloated stomach that looks like I could be pregnant, but I am not.

I don't have my health anymore, my earning power is gone, my allergies are ridiculous, my immune system is attacking itself and different foods started to smell vile to me again. It took me a while to realise there was a problem and I wasted some good meats by throwing them out thinking they were off. It was only when I was about to throw another good piece of meat out and a loved one asked why as the meat was fine, that it became apparent that it was just my sense of smell that was once again out of whack just as it had been during my pregnancy.

I think that's it. So to those who have given birth, look back at your pregnancy and you may get an idea of how your menopause might be. Knowing what I know now I am thinking my hormones didn't realign fully after my pregnancy, as this is when a few more allergies appeared. Not to the extent that they have since Ms Menopause knocked, but it seems that it all started back then after giving birth. If I had had the knowledge I now have after the birth of my daughter I would have had my hormones tested then.

It baffles me as to why we are not taught more about our bodies' hormones when they are the two main players in a woman's life, all the way from puberty to menopause. I don't know. I read articles where scientists are finding that certain autoimmune diseases are more gender based and affect women more than men. These scientists are doing studies to work it out which of course involves lots of money. My first thought is, "You are joking aren't you?" Just give me a quick call and I will tell you why women are more affected by autoimmune diseases. It's our oestrogen and progesterone. Our hormone system is interwoven with our immune system and when Ms Menopause comes a knocking, the loss of most of our estrogen and the loss of all of our progesterone has such a devastating effect on our immune system that it can create certain autoimmune diseases. But what do I know, I am just a girl in the world. Yeah, the mind just boggles.

It is also making sense now as to why I have an allergy with our dog that we brought home in 1998. Why didn't I have allergies to dogs throughout my life before I gave birth to my daughter? I reckon it is all hormone based. I don't think my menstrual cycles were long enough on a month-to-month basis to bring out my allergies even though my oestrogen and progesterone were being affected. I don't think the nine months of being pregnant, even though the allergy to dogs and such appeared, was long enough to do real damage, and also keep in mind our estrogen and progesterone step back into line, or are supposed to, after pregnancy.

I do know now that due to menopause and the loss of my oestrogen and progesterone, which my body will never again produce naturally, I have these allergies. This is also the reason my immune system is attacking itself.

I sit here and type thinking that really I don't have any allergies! What the...? Ok, I did have allergies to certain grasses and cats when I was a kid, but that was it. My immune system is purely the way it is because of the loss of those two hormones. As for the childhood asthma, which I grew out of, I never had to be hospitalized because of it, and I don't recall being on "puffers" to alleviate it either. So my childhood asthma must have been very minor.

All these allergies could have been avoided and would have been nonexistent if I'd had more knowledge when I first met Ms Menopause. Actually even if I'd had more knowledge after giving birth to the daughter. Yeah a few thoughts are gathering now. I only became allergic to penicillin after giving birth. To be fair, I don't recall needing penicillin before my pregnancy, and let's remember I could eat and drink whatever I wanted. I wonder now if this is why some younger women are dealing with Ms Menopause so early.

Some musings: Could it be that after their pregnancies, their oestrogen and progesterone also didn't align fully? In a case of a younger woman dealing with menopause before the average age, maybe their hormones were a lot less than mine therefore throwing them into early menopause, whereas with me the non-alignment of my hormones after pregnancy only affected me with a few allergies, but of course now in menopause I get the whole lot! So yeah, very interesting. Perhaps by getting our hormones checked after birth and getting onto BHRT then, we could avoid a lot of suffering.

I just had a thought! Does that mean that if I had been aware of this, I would have had my hormones checked back then and if needed, which obviously it was, I would have started BHRT which would have meant that there was no need to have all those desensitization injections, no need for Ms Menopause to be so debilitating, no need to lose my earning power and my friendships and the main one, that there would have been no need for the hardship all of this has caused my loved ones? AND I would still have my front tooth in my head? Oh getting to the tooth soon. Wow that is pretty massive. I am feeling a bit overwhelmed, I need time to ponder it so let's move on.

Chapter 32

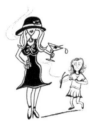

IT NEVER RAINS BUT IT POURS

I use this expression quite a lot in our family circle. It means basically that situations tend to follow each other in rapid succession or we have lots to deal with all at the same time. Like the time in 2004 when my sister was in the adult hospital still fighting her leukaemia, and at the same time my daughter was in the children's hospital across the road having an operation on the tendon in her right foot. Sadly, as I've mentioned, my sister lost her fight not long after that hospital stay. Fortunately my daughter, after weeks in a wheelchair, recovered from her ordeal. Right after that, our dad found out he had bowel cancer and after much love and care, in 2006 we also lost this beautiful man. So that is what I mean when I say it never rains but it pours in our family.

After seeing the endocrinologist, and before seeing my new allergist, I was again admitted to hospital. This admittance though, starts with the daughter. Now my daughter had quite a few problems with asthma as a child, but as she got older, and even though she has had to still deal with it at times in her young adult life, (she is twenty-one now) the asthma attacks were few and far between.

The daughter had decided to defer her studies and obtain a full time job. The first two weeks of training were done at one office building, then they were moved into their work places in a building in the city which was being refurbished. The girl was enjoying this new job; her only complaint was that the new training room in the new building was hot and stuffy as the air conditioning wasn't working properly. Two weeks into this job my daughter started to get sick. She became so sick that she needed a few days off after only being there for five weeks, which really upset her. The daughter picked up then crashed again, needing to be admitted to hospital. She was so sick they were thinking at one stage she needed to go to ICU (Intensive Care Unit).

I am watching this all go down and as her mum, knew that this was a different pattern to the past. The daughter, knowing I wasn't well, didn't want me to go and see her but as her mamma, and as unwell as I was, there was no way my daughter was going to be in hospital without me being there for her. I was very fortunate as loved ones would drop me off and pick me up, so I didn't have to worry about parking or walking too far.

They sent her home after a few days on two types of antibiotics not really knowing what was wrong with her. To cut a long story short, (am I capable of that?) the daughter got back to work but was still not well. In the eight weeks she was at this job she'd had about two weeks off in total and in the end had to quit, which was very disheartening for her.

After having a week to "get better," the girl got another job and feeling a little stronger, started her new position which was closer to home. It didn't take long for her to crash and burn again. Once when I picked her up from this job - yep we are now down to one car between all of us - the girl came out crying. Now the daughter has always had a good work ethic, but now she was coming out of work as it was a struggle for her to get through one shift. After giving her a hug I reassured her that we would get on the top of this.

I know my daughter, and this pattern of being sick then well then sick was just different, and I always had a niggling suspicion that this all had to do with that building in the city, but every time I mentioned the words "Legionnaire's disease" my daughter would get annoyed. We came home and the girl lay down on the lounge. I wrote down all her symptoms for our family doctor and at the bottom of the list I wrote, "I am her mum, this pattern is different," then I wrote Legionnaire's disease as well. I rang and booked her an appointment that same day, which is unusual in itself to get an appointment just hours before going, it was just fortunate that he had a spare slot.

Before going in, my daughter read the list and said in quite an annoyed way, "Don't say Legionnaires to him mum!" I told her that the list was for me to read out to him. Ok, so in with the doctor, I told him what was going on, read out her symptoms and as soon as he heard one particular symptom, without one word from me, he stated that it could be Legionnaire's disease. I wish I had a photo of the daughter's face when she looked at me after he said Legionnaires. Priceless. The doctor then asked if he could look at my list and sent the daughter off for blood tests there and then.

Blood tests came back in time and confirmed that yes, the daughter did indeed have a strain of legionnaires called *legionalla pneumonia infection*. The girl then had to be put on super dooper antibiotics and had to explain to the boss at her new job that she wasn't able to come back to work for four weeks. Thankfully they kept her job for her. The health department has been advised but as yet we have heard nothing definite as to where my daughter caught this.

I know, and I say it with much confidence, that it's that building. I looked into this disease myself and saw that the time frame between the daughter working in this building and her starting to get sick fits. The daughter is back up and running now and back at her workplace, but all in all the girl missed approximately eight weeks of pay because of this, but her health is more important. Although the girl is back at work I see that her health is still not as it was so I booked her in to see my BHRT doctor to see if we can get her back on top of her health naturally. Yes I made this booking for the daughter after I finally saw him, which I talk about later.

I get a little disappointed in myself for allowing the daughter to suffer for so long. I told her that will be the last time I let anyone stop me from following my intuition and my gut feeling. I said this looking straight at the daughter.

So when we got her home from hospital I started to crash and burn myself which annoyed me as I have always be the one who cares for my family. When my daughter who was picking up, thank god, asked me how I was, all I could say, with a heavily congested chest was, "I just want to die." I know it's a dramatic statement but I could hardly breathe. I tried to soldier on but we had to end up calling an ambulance. When they turned up they put an oxygen mask on me and whisked me off to hospital.

I was only in for the night and some of the next day, but my wonderful bro took a sickie from work to come up and make sure I was all right. There was no point in anyone else coming up as I was so bloody sick, and I had told the daughter not to come up as I wanted her to keep healing. It was horrible. I had to explain to them about my allergies and that I was allergic to penicillin blah blah blah.

I remember sitting there and, through an oxygen mask, asking the doctor in front of me how long it would be before I felt human again. Once again they were not too sure what was wrong with me. I did mention that the daughter had just been admitted a few days ago, and I am pretty sure I mentioned my suspicions about the building. I also mentioned that one of the daughter's bosses had just come back from overseas and had to have a week off due to food poisoning, but I was so sick I couldn't even say for sure that I did mention it. I was given antibiotics and asked the next day if I felt I could go home. Of course it was, "Yes please!" I still wasn't well but they also upped my steroids, so I knew as long as I could breathe I could be at home.

I have, since then, been tested for Legionnaire's disease but it came back negative. As my doctor said, I just have to be a bit more careful with the way my allergies and immune system are at present as it allows me to catch "bugs" more easily, and normal little sniffles can turn into much bigger things. I have supported family and friends on many occasions when they have been in hospital but not once have I ever been affected like that by all the bugs lurking in hospital corridors.

On seeing my doctor after all this, he said that it was really great that I picked up on what was happening to the daughter. It was nice of him to say, but I had to thank him and tell him that it was because he listened and acted on it that my daughter is ok now. And I really meant it. Doctors need to listen more. Yes they have done the years of study but they need to put their egos to the side and understand that we lay people are living it.

So again much gratitude to the best doctor in the universe! Oh and gee thanks to the nurse with the loud voice who was checking my details when I was admitted to hospital. This is how it went:

Nurse: You are blah blah, your date of birth is blah blah, you live at blah blah, and on about allergies.

Me: [Nodding and thinking "A bit loud don't you think?" This next bit was a wee bit "Geez almighty" to me]

Nurse: You are fifty-two and never been married.

Me: [Nodding and thinking "Geez do you think you could have screamed that out a little louder? Not only have you given a potential creep in another bed all my details but now he thinks I am a spinster and I live alone! So much for confidentiality. Let him know I have zilch in my bank account and that I am allergic to housework. That should turn him off. The oxygen mask is on my mouth love, not over my bloody ears!"]

It gave me a sense of all those wonderful eighty year olds who get screamed at because everyone just assumes that because they are in the later chapters of their lives, they are all deaf.

I personally haven't a problem with the fact that I have never married. I could have but just couldn't do it. I have never walked around in my life thinking there was something wrong with me or that I am missing anything because I am not married. I did say earlier though that I always felt like my fifties were going to be my best years. I also always had a feeling that I would get married in my fifties but as we all know, so far my fifties have been taken over by Ms Menopause.

Not that there is anything wrong with being a spinster. Did you know the name came from women who use to spin wool as a job in the 1300s? It was one of the few jobs available to women back then where they could earn their own dollars and live independently without needing the support of a male's wage. Apparently in the 1700s it changed into the meaning we know today.

Actually, if it wasn't for the daughter, just like my inner other-life transvestite (yes you will read about that later), I think I have an inner other-life spinster in me too. Long gone are the days when the whole concept of being a spinster was totally different. The majority of spinsters in today's world are independent women who choose not to marry or who were not prepared to take second best and think, "Something is better than nothing," but their lives are no less fulfilled than those who have married.

Spinsters have the freedom to do exactly what they want and they have the freedom to "do" whomever they want. They will never go through a horrible marriage or have to have a messy divorce. The money they have is all their own, to be spent exactly how they want. People might argue that at the end of spinsters' days they might not have anyone to care or be there for them. Well I say, look around, there are a lot of elderly people who have families but who still spend the end of their days alone. Anyway, I never had my daughter so that she could take on the role of being my carer when I get old! In this life I was blessed to have my daughter and I couldn't imagine my life without her love in it or the love I have for her. Being a mum gave me purpose and has been the most fulfilling, rewarding and best job I have ever been given. It has helped to have a wonderful daughter as well. If people ask me am I or have I ever been married I say, "Not yet." A mate of mine once said, "At least you can say you have never had to deal with a divorce." Ha! I liked it! Over the years though, I have always thought I would rather be without a husband than without a child. Husbands can come and go. My child is the core of me and I am very proud to be her mum.

I must say though, I have met many wonderful people with wonderful marriages, with and without children. For me my life just panned out the way it was meant to and to be honest I am very content with it. Oh and just to clarify, if I never meet that bloke, that will be ok because I know as soon as I get away from the strangle hold of Ms Menopause I am going to live my life to the fullest again. I have just never been the type to need a man to complete me, as wonderful as are most of the men I have had and still have in my life. Oh okay, maybe once in my lifetime I may have found a man who I felt completed me, you know, "you ying, me yang," but as it turned out, it was not to be.

Chapter 33

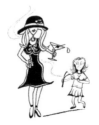

MY SHINY AND NEW ALLERGIST

The time was getting closer to seeing my new allergist, but of course something else happened a few days before. Throughout menopause and due to the loss of estrogen, we can have gum problems and loss of teeth. My front tooth – yes my front tooth! - was feeling quite sore and I could feel it was getting wiggly. One day it just popped out of my head into my hand. Oh yes indeed! Really Ms Menopause? My *front* tooth? With only days until I see my shiny and new allergist? Now of course a back tooth would not be an option for Ms Menopause and as I looked at that tooth sitting in the palm of my hand a whole "Bag Lady" scenario just played out in my head. Ms Menopause tried morphing me into the male version of myself which I have mentioned, and now, because she couldn't, she is trying another tactic!

ACT 1: I take off into the horizon pushing my shopping trolley with the bag of stuff I own. I have my bag lady outfit on held together with a rope belt. I have a material daisy and stem hat on, which "be-bops" side to side as I walk. Geez almighty! My *front* tooth? I know it's not a

190

biggie as I can fix it and I have dealt with bigger things. Hell, we even had fun with it, you know photos and poses, but I am days away from seeing my new allergist. I have stood in front of the mirror and tried to talk to see if the missing tooth won't be noticed. I tell you all it's near impossible. Oh well what can you do? I wonder if the new allergist understands mime.

I apologize if I offended anyone with the above. I am always grateful for the roof over my head, the shoes on my feet, the food in my belly and the love I have around me. I know compared to many I am very blessed but honestly, when I was staring at that tooth in my hand my mind just played out the whole bag lady scene!

The day came to see him. I told him I was there for a second opinion, I explained the tooth, and then we got down to business. He took my history and other information. He was quite surprised that, considering the state of my skin, the first allergist had been doing skin prick tests on me. I then asked his advice on my thoughts about it all being caused by menopause and how I didn't think we'd get a good result with my allergies until we got to a baseline with my hormones. His reply was, "You could be right." I also asked him if he was ok with his reports being released. He said he didn't care where they went. Yay, I thought as trying to get a report out of the first allergist was like trying to pull hens' teeth.

I was sent off to have blood tests done plus a few others, and was to come back soon for the results. This new allergist also said that due to the long-term use of steroids, my gums could be affected. Ok so is it my estrogen or the steroids? Oh it's a double whammy, of course it is! He also said that my adrenal glands would not be functioning properly and the results I have received in the past would have given false readings due to the steroids I've been on. Well there you go. I always knew my adrenal glands were sick from the moment I stumbled onto them in my research. I know my doctor had previously told me that steroids suppress the adrenal glands but I didn't put two and two together until now. I went off and had eight vials of blood taken plus a little extra to be put onto glass slides. The new allergist also put me on a daily antibiotic to stop infection.

Whilst on the allergy topic, for those of you who are menopausal and who have your nails done, you can have reactions to the glue and chemicals used in applying them. Also hair dyes can cause a reaction at this time of your life.

In amongst all the other thoughts I had been having for a while about how my funds are drying up, and due to the first allergist not giving a rat's ass and being incompetent, the people who are controlling my pocket money are taking a lot longer than expected to give me more. My loved ones have been wonderful helping financially but why should they have to do that? They work damn hard for their money.

I realized that to get my health back to where I am "me" again, I needed funds to do so. Being sick is not just exhausting, it is expensive. I didn't want to have to wait for the people who are controlling the funds I am entitled to, to decide whether I am still sick or not. Anyway I don't know where all this is heading or even how much time I have until I just "pop." I don't want to have to wait longer than needed just due to lack of funds. So all I could think about was….

Chapter 34

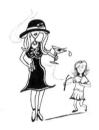

CENTRELINK AGAIN! WITH A HAPPY ENDING

I had decided that my family had done enough for me financially and that I needed to talk to Centrelink again. I have not received anything from them since December 2012. Now this also means all the medications I have needed have been more expensive as well. The Centrelink funds though came to me in July 2013. Our combined family funds have been ok, but it's time to take the stress off. Also I feel a wee bit stronger, so I might be able to string a sentence together this time without crying.

I sent them an email through their website. I received a letter stating I was to send the required paperwork to them and I had until the 9th of August to re-engage with them. I sent a letter through the post asking what paper work was needed. I also sent copies of my doctor's bits and pieces. I heard nothing. The 9th of August came and went. I went to my doctor to get another three month Centrelink certificate. I went to Centrelink with the daughter, as again she wanted to support me. The daughter was getting very over the way I have been treated at times. I am too, but I still haven't got the voice I used to have.

We lobbed up to our local Centrelink office. When I handed the guy I was dealing with my certificate he said, "What's this for?" I said, "To get money." I then asked him about the letter I had sent to the manager of this branch, as she had been the one who responded to my original email. You know what he did next? He just shrugged his shoulders.

Well have you seen those Current Affairs shows on TV that show people going wild at their Centrelink offices? I could tell the daughter was starting to get agitated, so I told her not to worry. His attitude was horrible so I said, almost in a whisper, "Your attitude towards people who are not well is terrible. You need to have more compassion, especially when you are the front line guy and we have to deal with you." It was nearly a whisper but it was my voice!

His attitude did change after that and he was a bit more likeable. He explained that the letter had not been received at their office and I would have to make a call to Centrelink to get linked up again. Yeah I know, we are already at Centrelink but I have to go home and call Centrelink. Go figure. So off we went and as soon as we walked out the door my daughter and I roared with laughter. I told you we have a weird sense of humour, and we also laughed about how I was getting worried that she was going to pick stuff up and throw it through the window or start to burn the place down. I just don't want to have my fifteen minutes of fame on TV when I am not well and not looking my best. Vain I know.

I'm at home on the phone. The first person asks what payment I am going on - true story.

Me: I have no idea, that is why I was told to ring you.

Him: So you don't know what payment you are going on? Is it Newstart or Disability?

Me: No idea mate, you need to sort it, look at my records. I was just in at the "Blah blah" office and they said I had to ring you.

See? Nobody knows where to place the suffering menopausal woman.

The first person transferred me to a second person and here starts my happy ending. I went through it all with her.

Her: So they did nothing for you at that office?

Me: No and to be truthful, from what I have heard it happens nine out ten times that they send people off to call you. Oh and also the guy was rude and I had to put his attitude in check.

Her: Ok so let's get this sorted, what is the reason you are sick and have been unable to work?

Me: I am menopausal and have been dealing with it since 2010.

As soon as menopause was mentioned she said that she too was having a rough time of it, crying at work, feeling anxious and not being able to work some days. I am very sorry to hear that this woman was struggling and I felt like I had found a kindred spirit. After getting some history from me this woman then booked me an appointment back at the original office to get my payment set up. Before we finished we had a bit of a chinwag about Ms Menopause. She said from her experience and a few of her friends' experiences, that doctors seem to think steroids and antidepressants are the way to treat the menopausal woman. When she said this it was music to my ears, it's just nice to know it's not only me! Thank you wonderful Centrelink employee for getting this sorted for me. I am still a bit confused about having to pay back the November payment, but I will sort that out later.

So a few days later off I went to my appointment. I was dreading it. The young girl was respectful and set me up on Newstart. I asked if this meant I would be contacted by employment agencies again. She said yes as they like to keep us linked to them. I then said, "I have a doctor's certificate here stating I cannot work. I am not well enough to be hounded by employment agencies again. It is just extra stress to deal with when I just want to concentrate on trying to get better. If you don't attend these appointments they cancel your payment and that will happen to me as I won't be attending them."

Yes apparently even if your doctor tells them you cannot work, they can and still do set it up for employment agencies to contact you. What *is* that? Oh still waiting for my happy ending? Believe it or not it is coming. The young girl then said an appointment was being set up for me to have an Employment Services Assessment. Ok, so all that I had just said went in one ear straight out the other. I thought great, I am finally getting my voice back and I just dug a deeper hole for myself without any help from Ms Menopause at all. Lucky that she was still slothing at home, she would have been delighted to see all this go down. Unfortunately her troops, aka symptoms, go everywhere with the menopausal woman so no doubt they will all report back to her and get a good hearty laugh out of it. Laugh away, let's see who is laughing when the time comes for me to pack all your bags and kick you back out onto the kerb!

I was then given a pamphlet to explain the next appointment I was to attend. We then finally got to the part about my payment. What I didn't know was that my payment had been backdated to the date of my original email to them via their website. Wow! I didn't know that was coming, and I was due another payment at the end of the week. So now I had enough of "me own dollars" to help a bit more with household bills and to pay back those dollars that were used to see my new allergist. I walked out of there thanking the universe but still not looking forward to the other appointment I had to come back for in a week.

Chapter 35

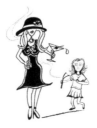

BACK TO THE SPECIALISTS

M y first port of call was to book in with the BHRT doctor. Once there I was told he had closed his books until next month! So close and yet so far when I didn't have the funds, and now with funds in hand I had to wait until next month before I could even try and get to see him! Feck! Feck! Feck! I went home feeling deflated and exhausted, but when I really thought about it I knew next month wasn't too far away so I rang them back to see if I could call them early on the 1st of the new month:

Me: I was just down there and was told Dr's books are closed until next month.

Voice: I don't know why you were told that, who told you that?

Me: I don't know, a young girl at reception.

Voice: Let me know what you need to see him for and I will have a chat to the doctor and ring you back.

Me: Menopause blah blah want to trial BHRT blah blah.

Voice: Ok leave it with me and I will get back to you.

Lucky I just didn't sit back on my laurels. Come on phone, ring, and please let it be good news. Well the phone did ring and it was good news. An appointment was made and I was so happy! I yam what I yam and I yam elated! The name I had been carrying around on that piece of paper was getting closer to being a real person.

I am tired though. Just getting up and through my days is enough to tire me out, let alone getting to all my appointments at times. I am hoping that all the tiredness and exhaustion will all be worth it when I get through all of this.

It was time to go back to my new allergist for results. As I went up to the receptionist desk and told her who I was, I was asked which one I was as the allergist was seeing two Jennifer Townsends. I tell you now it made my blood run cold. I said in a joking way but fully meaning it, "So he is fully aware that there are two of us?" The response was, "Of course." That was sorted and I was confident that in any dealings I had with them, as long as I introduced myself as JT from Blahblah, a bit like J-LO from the block, all would be fine. I know some may think I am overreacting a bit, but we're not talking about two people with the same name who put in a pizza order at the same time and there is a chance of the order getting mixed up, if you get my drift.

Anyhoo, in I went. My chest x-ray came back ok. My bone density test came back ok and I haven't got lupus, but I wasn't expecting what came next. It turns out I have an over active immune system which is attacking itself and has caused the inflammation and the severe atopic dermatitis. I'd had a niggling feeling for a while that all was bigger than just my allergies, and right then it was confirmed. I also said to him, "Whether you agree with me or not, I still believe this all stems back to menopause." His response was, "I don't disagree with you." Then nearly in a whisper he said, "It could have something to do with your oestrogen." I had my head bowed as he said this but I looked at him and said, "And progesterone."

198

So there you go, finally someone in the medical world, although still in a roundabout and non-committed way, had said that I could be right; that my allergies wouldn't be fixed until we got to a baseline with my hormones, and that he didn't disagree with me that this could all be due to menopause, and that the illness I was now facing could have something to do with my oestrogen. It is unfortunately a little too late though as far as I am concerned.

The allergist then explained two medications that I had to choose from that he felt I needed to take. I had two weeks to choose between Azathioprine and Cyclosporin. It was also explained that I would have to be closely monitored and blood tests would have to be taken weekly. It turns out both of these medications are used to stop rejection of organs in transplant patients.

He also went through some of the possible side effects: my kidney function could be affected, my number of white cell counts which are needed to fight infection could drop, my number of platelets which help to stop bleeding could also drop. They can have effects on my liver, pancreas, blood pressure and increase the risk of sun cancers. They can cause tremors of the hands, rashes and the list of many goes on.

The allergist printed out copies of patient information on these two medications so I could read up on them at home before I made my choice. He also explained that not all of these side effects may happen, but they were all possible common, less common or rare side effects. Yeah you reckon, I thought. After everything I have been through I'm thinking that I will be hit with each and every one of those side effects, and knowing me I will most probably create a few more to add to their already "scary as" list!

As he was filling out a Centrelink certificate for me, yes I had that appointment the next day and I thought they might actually believe that I am sick if I had a certificate from this new allergist, I flicked through and read that one of the medications can cause thicker and darker hair on our face. I said, "Oh fabulous," out loud. When he questioned me I said, "Well this one says we can get thicker and darker hair on our face, but that's fine as that will go nicely with the moustache menopause gives us." As he laughed, I thought, "Why are you laughing, I wasn't trying to be funny I was just stating the facts!"

I tell you all now, I walked out of there feeling pretty damn sorry for myself. So this is what it has come to. I am a menopausal woman in the 21st century and Ms Menopause has been allowed to turn me into a middle aged woman with a mental disorder who is dealing with other symptoms of hers and now also dealing with a serious illness which needs serious medication. I would like to say that Ms Menopause is at home packing her bags and thinking, "Well my job here is done, let's move onto the next one," but I've got a feeling she isn't going anywhere until I am "done and dusted."

You know I missed that bit. The bit about how women are living in old age with illnesses that stem back to Ms Menopause. The bit I missed was, I am now living with an illness in my middle age and I may not even get to my old age! We have to always remember that the medical world is allowing Ms Menopause to do this to the menopausal woman.

Yeah the walk back to my car after getting all this from the allergist was a very slow one. I felt, even more so for this moment, like a "dead woman walking." But, oh yes the good old but, even before I got to my car Plan B had popped into my head and that is BHRT, and I had made a decision on those two medications as I was still buckling up my seat belt. I just needed time to read up on the information I was given, have a moment to compose myself, put my brave voice on and then gather the loved ones to discuss my decision.

The decision I made was that I wasn't going on either of those medications. I believe I would be in a bigger mess than I am already in now if I took either of those. I am not doing it tougher, and I certainly am not doing that to my family. My quality of life would be even less and I would need more care. The many side effects that can happen are too severe. I know I have days now where I don't function properly but I know those meds would make it worse. The allergist said that some of the side effects can be reversed down the track but I forgot to ask him how. I am guessing that the attempted reversal will be with other super dooper drugs. Blow that! My loved ones read the material on the meds and they supported me in my decision. I did have another quiet chat to the daughter later to make sure she was ok. My beautiful daughter said, "I support you in whatever decision you make and mum I really believe you have made the right one."

I understand I just made a life decision. I am under no illusion that BHRT may be the answer to my health problems but I reckon I have a better fighting chance doing it my way. I will say though, that with hope and faith I actually do have a quiet confidence in BHRT, but how am I supposed to shout out all its virtues if I don't use it myself?

If all fails I have to go out as close as I can to being me. I also had a chat to my best mate away from my loved ones and said that if it is my time, I want to make sure she plays "I'm Not Okay" and "Welcome to the Black Parade" by My Chemical Romance at that thing people have when they pass over. I feel really content with my decision and to be honest it wasn't even a hard one to make. Now I just need to get the support from all those I am dealing with in the medical world.

As satisfied as I was about the decision I had made, I did have a moment of thinking pretty deeply into it. I went to bed thinking that maybe it was just meant to be that my time had come. Instead of fighting so hard to be healthy and stay alive, maybe it was time to accept it all and start preparing to die. I can tell you also that at the end of your days there is a sense of the real, deep love you have, and for me it was only a handful of family and friends that I thought about. I just had to trust in the universe to watch over them if I am meant to go. Oh wait a minute; I could bloody watch over them myself! It was quite a weird feeling. It was as if acceptance had come and I felt lighter. I wasn't scared, I just felt at peace, and I slipped into sleep feeling like this.

201

Well the first thing that popped into my head as soon as I woke up was "WALK." True! I got out of bed got changed, told my family member I was going to start walking again and so I did! Ha, don't know where that came from, well I reckon I do. I walked for about thirty minutes. It was slow, tiresome and my body hurt but I did it. Oh ok I had to ring a family member to come and get me as I knew I wasn't going to make it back, but I did half of it! I walked like this for a few days then tired out. But I have started to try and walk twice now, so I will try again soon. I really felt better mentally and emotionally after these walks. My head felt clearer and I was ready to fight for my survival again. I have stated I am not scared to die. To be honest if I didn't have love ones I don't think the fight for my survival and just to "be" would be so important. Yes, there is nothing like the love we have for those who make us want to be around for the long haul. And thank you to my loved ones who have passed over before me for getting me out of that bed and walking. I knew it was you guys, I love you all!

Now I had to do the rounds regarding my decision. So as not to leave anything out I want to get through this time in one fell swoop. I am not writing in real time, I am still catching up and it really tires me out to have to relive all this again. All of the following sounds like it has happened in one week, but it was actually took place over several weeks so:

Centerlink, then my doctor, then the BHRT doctor, then the BHRT doctor again, then my new allergist, then last but not least, my doctor again.

The appointment went well with Centrelink. They are giving me a payment for a year. Of course it needs assessing as other pocket money comes through, and they are stopping all employment agencies from contacting me so that I can concentrate on trying to get better. At the end I gave the girl the allergist's certificate and it made me realize that this decision was made without his input. Hmm, interesting. A week later I received a health care card. A week later I received another letter stating that it was cancelled which left me thinking what now? But reading further on it said that my health card was going to be replaced with a pension card. Okay. All good, thank god. Oh and to the young girl from Centrelink who set up this appointment, I know now that what I had said didn't just go in one ear and out the other so thank you to both of you.

It did make me wonder why the decision to do this for me was only made now, considering I have been just as sick all the way through, and the decision was made on viewing my doctor's certificate which had the same detailed information which was given to them in 2012. This new decision made by Centrelink was without the new allergist's certificate as that was only attached as a "we will put that in your records" afterthought. Yeah, very interesting.

Then I was off to see my doctor. The first question I asked him was had he received the allergist's report and the authority to release it? I had already emailed previously trying to get this to my doctor. He had received the report and had it in a white envelope waiting for me but couldn't release it to me as he needed the allergist's ok in writing. Fair enough I say. My doctor needs to protect himself; he has a family and mouths to feed. I told him of my decision not to go on those medications the allergist wanted me to, and explained that I wanted to try BHRT and asked if he would support me for three months. He wasn't too happy about my decision but said yes, he would support me. I then went home and again emailed my allergist in regard to the authority. I need this report to be sent to those who dish out my pocket money.

Now the time had come to finally meet my BHRT doctor. This bloke called out my name and there in front of me was the name on my piece of paper which finally had materialized into a real human being. The first question I asked him was, "Are you a doctor who specializes in BHRT?" Yes he was, but he was an "integrated" doctor. He works with western medicine if needed but also with natural therapies and Chinese medicine. He explained that western medicine had only been around for 100 years or so but the natural medicines have been around for centuries. I then said, "So you are not a normal doctor then?" When he said that it could be put like that I said, "Well then that would make you a special doctor."

I also asked him two other questions before we got into it all and they were:

Are there natural steroids? He told me there were adrenal herbs, ok so I will look into them later, and:

Had he heard of the book called "What Your Doctor May Not Tell You About Menopause" by Dr John Lee? He answered yes; it was the first book he read when he had decided to go into his chosen medical field.

Wow! You know I could have kissed him. We had a quick chat, I told him about the meds I was not going to go on, and that I wanted to try BHRT again under his guidance. He then suggested that my doctor and allergist would not be too happy about the decision I had made. You know all I could think to say back to him was, "Well that's just bad luck, it's my life!"

Through it all it was really uplifting to talk to a doctor who thinks out of the box. Mental note to self: you are not his only patient. He is not there exclusively for you. No! You cannot take him home to keep chatting and to be able to ask him questions as they pop into your head while he is stirring the bolognaise sauce for the al dente spaghetti. Okay self. I get it!

He sent me off for blood tests to check my hormones, and a container to wee into, as he wanted to do some special testing with it. He had asked if he could ring the allergist to get more of a handle on what was going on with me. I said yes and was happy that he wanted to. The only request I had was that he didn't tell the allergist of my decision. I wanted to do that myself face to face.

I walked out of there elated and with hope again by my side. All bloods were taken and soon enough I was back with my BHRT doctor. He had spoken to my new allergist and he informed me that the allergist had only intended to put me on one tenth of the strength of those medications that are used to stop rejection of organs in transplant patients. Oh really I thought, the allergist had not conveyed that snippet of very vital information to me. Not that it matters. If I have to be monitored closely and have weekly blood tests done whilst on one-tenth strength of this medication… well my prayers go out to those who have no choice and need the full strength.

The blood results show that my oestrogen was low and I had zero progesterone in my body. My testosterone was fine and strong which didn't surprise me as I always felt like I was part "man." I had always joked with mates that in another life I reckon I would have been a transvestite! Oooh do you remember Tim Curry who played a transvestite in "The Rocky Horror Picture Show?" Oh my god, it was the only time in my whole life that I had actually lusted after another human being in high heels! He was absolutely gawjuzzz! Maybe that's why I blast "Sweet Transvestite," that he sang in that movie, in my car at times. Oh gawd, too much information? Sorry. Way too far off the track of Ms Menopause? Double sorry! What also didn't surprise me about the results was that my man hormone was kicking back taking it easy without a care in the world when my woman hormones were wilting and dying, screaming out for help!

The doctor thought that even though my estrogen was low, I had enough for now and got me started on the progesterone. He then gave me the script for the BHRT and I tell you, my doctor and I were not too far away from this new finely tuned script. He then said he would need to get the results of my urine done as soon as possible. The way he said it made me say, "You are scaring me now." His response was, "Well what you are dealing with is very serious and we need to get on top of it." You know, I know this is serious, I have known that for a long time,

205

it's just that when you hear the urgency in a doctor's voice, it makes it more real. So I walked out of there with my BHRT script in hand, leaving my urine sample with him, and with a heavy heart. I knew I was going to cry but I just wanted to get home first.

Then, as the glass doors opened for me to go to my car, we heard the screeching of car tyres and then heard a few loud bangs! A four-car smash had just happened in front of me at the traffic lights in front of the Centre. I stood there watching a woman get out of one of the cars and start fiddling with something in her back seat. She then pulled a baby out and just stood there in shock. A guy who was in a car a few behind her ran up to her and pointed over to the Medical Centre. It was horrible. One of the receptionists went out and guided her in. As they were walking in they were within touching distance from me and all I could do was look at this little limp angel. As they walked past the little one let out a cry, vomited and went limp again. Oh my god. It was terrifying. I wanted to go back in to see if the baby was ok but my whole being was starting to shake and I just needed to get home as the tears were now starting to fall.

As soon as I walked in my front door and was asked how it went, my sobs started coming from the bottom of my soul and I couldn't talk. All I could get out in a whisper and between sobs and my breaths was, "I just need a moment," and went into my bedroom and sobbed my eyes out. My poor family member was left thinking the worst, so as soon as I was able, I explained about the accident and the baby. I didn't tell them about the chat I had with my doctor, why worry my loved ones anymore than necessary? I did throw a prayer up to the universe to protect the little one, and we did hear about the smash on the news but nothing was mentioned about the baby so I am really hoping that means the little angel is ok.

While sitting at home on my pondering step I thought, "When did this all start to get serious?" Actually when did those involved start to take all this seriously? I know it has been serious for ages now; I am living it. But why only now are they seeing the urgency in it all. Centrelink is now playing nice and understands how serious it is. My new allergist knows how serious it is and my BHRT doctor understands the seriousness of it all as he scared the heck out me with the urgency in his voice! I'll tell you when they all started taking this seriously. It was when they had a different name to put to what I am dealing with. The name Menopause was never serious enough for them. God I am so angry with them all! They have allowed a natural part of a woman's life to turn into a serious illness and to strip me of pretty well all that I am and all that I had. Also, they have allowed my loved ones to go through all this too. I have to say it again as I have said many times and will continue to say many times, with earlier education and information which would give women options, none would have to suffer so severely through this natural phase of their lives. Who are the people making the decision that it is okay for a woman to suffer so much? Ok Jen, shake it off! Just shake it off! Well for now anyway.

It was time now to see my new allergist. It was a bit unnerving as I was driving in to see him. Here I was ready to say, "Yeah but no thanks," to an opinion given by a professional who is one of the best in his field. I really wanted his support but I knew if he wouldn't give it, nothing would change my decision. I also never forget that it is that mob, the Medical World, which got me into this mess in the first place by not taking Ms Menopause more seriously. I have to try and save myself because right now I'm not feeling that that mob is going to save me.

I went in and sat down after saying I was JT from Blahblah. It went well. I told him of my decision and he said the main thing was to try and get me to some state of wellness again. I told him that was what I was trying to do and those other meds he wanted me to choose from scared the hell out of me. I asked him if he would support me for three months. He wasn't ecstatic about my decision but I have his support. I don't see him again for a few months, but can head back earlier if need be. Imagine how much less ecstatic he's going to feel when he knows those meds are never going to pass my lips. I give them this time frame as I think it makes them feel better.

I also asked him if I was going to die. He was a bit surprised and he fumbled around a bit. I then asked him to just be honest and let me know. Well his mouth all of a sudden seemed to fill up with invisible marbles, so I thought I'd help him out by saying, "I know we are all going to die, I would just prefer it to be at eighty-four than at fifty-two." That was it. I walked away knowing that even though I didn't get the answer to that question, all was as it should be, for him and me. I was a little annoyed at myself for even asking the question, but from the dealings I have had with this mob I don't want them giving me a twenty-four hour notice of my passing over! Also it wasn't fair to put him in that position and if he had given me an answer I would have been annoyed at him for thinking he is God. Yeah all is as it should be. Not knowing is another win-win situation as far as I am concerned.

Oh and we also discussed my missing front tooth. Thanks to my immune system and the fact that my skin hasn't got good healing powers at the moment, I can't get any dental work done until I am sitting on 7mg of steroids, which by my calculation is February 2014. The reason is that we need to see if my adrenal glands will kick back in and produce their own natural steroids again. Fabulous! Oh well, it's a minor detail. I am actually getting used to it. I reckon it would be a great photo shoot if I also had the "Who from Whoville" look to go with it. I am not out in the world as I used to be, so for now I can live with it. I could just keep my mouth closed and no one would notice, but let's get real here, that just isn't going to happen!

Ok, I now have a support group around me in the medical world, which respects the decision I have made. I am in the driver's seat of my life, well that is until Ms Menopause decides to throw something else at me. I really hope I get myself to my healthy and happy ending safely. I must say that the new allergist has been wonderful. He did a hell of a lot more for me than the first allergist. I know he tried to do his best in "the box" he practices out of, but, with respect, that box just isn't big enough or good enough for me as a menopausal woman in the 21st century.

Also, to rehash old news, he didn't disagree with me regarding Ms Menopause, so these specialists know what is possible with the menopausal woman, but still comments are only made in a non-committed way, if they are made at all. Actually that is the most open that any medical person has been with me since 2010 and we are heading towards Christmas 2013 so yeah, I've got to try and save myself.

Ok, last but not least, I head back to my doctor. I had been feeling a little bit dizzier than normal so I needed to get that looked at. All was checked; blood pressure was a bit up and down but otherwise my doctor feels it could also be from coming down in the steroids, but as usual he keeps a good eye on me. Of course I asked if he had received the authorization from the allergist to release his report yet. His reply was no, not yet.

Ok I am way over this now and I think my doctor is too. I am bloody tired. No I am bloody exhausted. He rang while I was still there and got the authorization over the phone with a statement that the authority had been sent. Oh really? To who? Oh okay, I'm with you now. You actually sent it to Who at Whoville because it's not here! Anyhoo the big white envelope was handed to me and as my doctor was organizing tests he wanted me to do, I had a quick skim through the reports. One was the original visit and one was the review. Well guess what? At the top of the original visit report it had the wrong Jennifer Townsend's details on it. No joke! True! I know! I read back on stuff thinking, "You are joking aren't you?" Un-bloody-believable!

To be honest I am not surprised. I have had to deal with obstacle after obstacle just trying to survive and get my health back since *she* knocked on my door. I think I might add in a chapter called "The Menopause Conspiracy."

I showed my doctor and he said, "What are the chances of him seeing two of you with the same name and this one is only six months older than you." I actually think he found it quite amusing in a "no way you gotta be joking" way. All I could say was, "Yeah I know, I read her details and I bet she is having problems with menopause too." My doctor wasn't giving away any private information to me because I knew all about Jennifer Townsend, oh I mean the other me, before he did!

So phone calls were made again. Firstly my doctor rang them back, explained the error and was told it would be fixed and faxed shortly. I had no intention of leaving until those reports came with me. Twenty minutes later - nothing. My doctor's receptionist rang again for me and was told, with attitude, that it was being done. A further twenty minutes later - nothing. My doctor was in and out with patients and he could see I was still waiting, so I mouthed to him I was going outside to ring them myself.

Some days my voice is back, other days I know it's not, today though was a good "I have my voice back" day. I spoke to the girl at the allergist's office and told her again of the error and that I wanted it fixed asap as I was not leaving until I had them. I then headed back in to take my seat in the waiting room. Five minutes later a call came through to the main desk and as soon as I heard my name the receptionist gave me the phone. The voice on the other end could not see the problem and kept talking over me. The voice started reading my details out and I said, "That is the review." You could hear by the silence that she had finally found the error, so I said, "You see that now?" The voice didn't stay silent for long so I had to say, "If you would just let me speak for a moment, the content is correct, but it has the wrong Jennifer Townsend's details on it." With a quick assurance that it would be fixed and faxed now, all I could think of saying was, "Ok as I am not leaving without it, ta." Within a few minutes, it was faxed with the correct details, I thanked all who had been involved at my doctor's centre, and off I went and faxed it to where it needed to go. Bloody hell!

So there you go, my dizziness has gone but I'm telling you, my head is still spinning from that! I hope the other me is getting all her correct reports. I came home and read and re-read mine to ensure it was me. A bit scary actually. Some days when I am home I just stare out the window and think about it all. Not only am I dealing with my health issues but also with other stuff that should not be happening. I am constantly tired; I should be just resting and trying to heal without all this other crap going on around me.

I had just settled down at home thinking all is organized and I get time off from them all for a little while, but no. I rang my BHRT doctor's receptionist to get results for that urine test I had done and was advised that my BHRT doctor wants to see me earlier than planned regarding the results. Oh my god I am pregnant! Ha ha he he chuckle chuckle! No I'm not! Just threw that in to make sure you are not falling asleep while reading this! I wasn't due to see him for a while as I have started the BHRT again and just thought I could get the results over the phone, but no. Over it! And I'm sure you are all over it too! I think we all need a break from it all. I will get to that later. I want to talk about other stuff I have found that hopefully will help your journey so let's do that.

Chapter 36

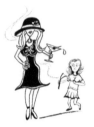

VITAMIN D AND COLLAGEN

When I was craving the sun and I found out I was vitamin D deficient, I didn't even relate this to Ms Menopause, I just knew I was deficient. My doctor had me do another blood test to check my Vitamin D again and the results showed that my levels were low. The normal range is 50-300, mine came back at 60. The doctors like us to be sitting at 100. This level of 60 must be a hell of a lot higher than it was in 2012 as I am not craving the sun anymore.

My doctor also told me that studies are being done that show low levels of Vitamin D can exacerbate allergies. Hmm, interesting. Of course I went off and investigated. Get yourselves nice and comfy because we all know there are no short stories for anything relating to "The Change," and it is no surprise to find out that this deficiency creates more than just allergy problems in menopausal women.

Losing estrogen through menopause leads to a change in our bone health. Estrogen increases the activity of the enzyme responsible for activating Vitamin D. When our estrogen decreases during menopause it causes a Vitamin D deficiency. This is a common problem. Vitamin

D is vital in bone building. It is also essential for the absorption of our calcium, which also increases bone health. Our bodies can be affected two fold if we are not getting enough vitamin D and calcium. With weak and brittle bones you then risk developing osteoporosis. This deficiency can also lead to muscle pain and/or weakness, depression and fatigue, sleep problems and mood swings. Studies show that this vitamin plays a core role in many of our body's processes and should be at the top of the list of concerns for menopausal women. It has been shown that vitamin D prevents heart disease, osteoporosis, diabetes, certain cancers, cardiovascular disease and also hypertension and weight gain. Once again knowledge brings prevention, which is your best defence.

I was also finding I was dealing with pain in my joints and muscles. I get sore ankles that feel like they should be swollen, but are not. My calf muscles and leg muscles get sore and feel like they're about to cramp but don't. My feet also get sore and get that cramping feeling which is really painful at times.

This is what I learnt from the *Amberen* Smart Choice for Menopause* site. I know this company sells a natural menopause treatment, but I don't know anything about it. If you do choose to use this product, look into it well, and if you have success, scream it out loud. The information I was finding on this site was simple and straight forward and without all the hocus pocus that surrounds menopause at times:

> Joint pain through menopause can make everyday tasks a challenge leaving you pained and drained. If joint pain is experienced one might assume it is due to "getting older." However, like many women in their 40s and 50s, your bone health and joint mobility may be profoundly affected by the hormonal shifts that take place during menopause. The medical term for this menopause joint pain is called "arthalgia". Interestingly enough, it is also known as "menopause arthritis."

Before I go on, I know I say nothing surprises me anymore in regard to Ms Menopause, but I must admit the "menopause arthritis" stunned me. Why? Well it is another part of menopause that is being blamed on old age. Are the majority of women living with arthritis in the later chapters of their lives living with it unnecessarily because it is actually a symptom of menopause? Could the majority of these women, with education and information, be living a happier and healthier life without arthritis? It goes on:

> Menopause arthritis can affect the back, knees, hips and extremities - this means the end part of a limb such as feet and hands - and some may find that fingers and wrists become sore. However during menopause, pain can be experienced throughout the other hundreds of joints.

Really? So that means I still have hundreds of joints to feel yet? Wow, thanks Ms Menopause! As the body contains more than 350 joints, pain could also be felt in the jaw, shoulder, elbows, neck, back, and the list just goes on.

Like many menopause symptoms, aching joints are caused by significant hormonal imbalances. Because oestrogen plays a role in preventing inflammation throughout the body, oestrogen deficiencies that occur in midlife can lead to inflamed painful joints. They say that testosterone levels can also fluctuate during menopause, leading to muscle loss that also strains joints. I haven't mentioned progesterone here as I have already covered it in some detail.

So there you go. To all those menopausal women who are being told their aches and pains are just due to getting old, it's a load of hogwash. It is caused by the hormonal imbalance we experience during this time of our lives. I always thought our fifties were supposed to be the new forties not the new 100s! Ok, mental note to self: I know I have always thought that I don't want to go out looking like mutton dressed up as lamb, well bugger that! If I get through this with health and self intact I will continue to dress however I want until my last breath, and as usual I will say, "If you don't like it, don't look!"

Yeah, so please god, let me get into my eighties healthy, happy and me. Please let me pass over with a bright outfit on, a full face of makeup, my usual crazy hair, dyed of course, what colour? Not too sure yet! And an empty chardy glass smashed on the ground next to my chair with my sixty year old toy boy touching up my lipstick before the loved ones arrive. Ta. Amen

Of course, after getting to know more about collagen, it too has become bigger than Ben Hur. I just thought collagens only purpose was to keep my face looking nice, how wrong can a girl be? I have noticed I have aged since my journey started with Ms Menopause, and I have also read many blogs where woman have seen the aging process in themselves happen faster in this period of their lives. I am hearing you sisters!

Collagen is all about giving our skin elasticity. Our skin's elasticity decreases with the loss of oestrogen which plays a part in the production of collagen. It is said that it is also due to the natural aging process. You know I get that, but from what I am reading and from what I am seeing when I look in my mirror, Ms Menopause also picks on your looks. Rebecca Booth MD wrote:

> Hormonal aging is one of the least known or discussed causes of wrinkling, dry skin and sagging skin.

And there is more! Collagen is like the body's glue. We lose elasticity in joints and in the walls of our arteries, and of course our vaginal system loses its elasticity too. Collagen helps with flexibility in our pelvic bones, which helps with vaginal delivery, for those who may need this information. The loss of collagen created by Ms Menopause can give you a gigantic bruise at the slightest bump. Collagen loss weakens blood vessels, there is less cushioning around the vessel wall, our skin becomes less resilient and it also helps to keep our eyes moist.

It connects and supports other body tissue e.g. skin, bone, tendons, muscles and cartilage.

And here I was thinking that collagen was in my body to keep my face and skin looking supple so my war paint, oops, makeup, would just glide easily over my collagen filled face. I actually got a bit scared when I found out that collagen is the body's glue. What? Am I going to end up a sack of skin with bones and other bits splattered on the ground calling out "Help Meeeeeee" like in the movie "The Fly" if I lose all of my body's glue? It just makes me shiver.

It is pretty scary to know that the loss of those two hormones, oestrogen and progesterone, plus a little testosterone loss, can do all this to us and yet we are not educated about it. I was talking to a nurse and she said that "they" think if we know all that could wrong with us in menopause that we will "just want to go on everything." Oh really, so the "they" in the 21st century think the menopausal woman is a simpleton do "they"? No, "they" got it wrong. If I had information and the available options at the beginning of my journey, I would have been able to make an intelligent, informed decision regarding my health and wellbeing. I ended the conversation by saying, "But they are letting menopause turn into an illness for women." Every time I speak to this nurse I keep forgetting to ask her who "they" are. Got to remember next time to ask. You know what I reckon? I reckon "they" know there is a lot of power in our ovaries.

Suzanne Somers was an actress who is now in her 60s and is still wonderfully healthy and gorgeous. Suzanne has been slammed by some in the medical world for the books she has written on menopause. She lays the blame for the criticism she gets from doctors partially on the fact that some of the medical experts have connections to pharmaceutical companies which, as we know, are profitable businesses. Suzanne states she is not a scientist, she is a layperson who is passionately interested in preserving quality of life, and is appalled by the lack of information we have about menopause. Good on you Suzanne, don't let these doctors or the medical community intimidate you. Suzanne is giving women safer choices than HRT. As a layperson, she attends alternative medical conferences and this wonderful woman is trying to find answers for all those dealing with Ms Menopause. She will continue to be slammed by the medical community. Why? Because it's all about money and profit.

This is just another example of the medical community trying to smear a woman who is looking for the truth and safe therapies for women. I don't know if your daily routine would suit, or even be affordable for, the average woman, but we are definitely on the same page with wanting education, truth, safer therapies and bringing menopause out into the open.

I do get though, your daily routine of sixty odd vitamin supplements and bio identical hormone creams. From what I gather, many think your daily routine is extreme, but with all your knowledge about how big Ms Menopause really is and how she affects our bodies in so many ways, well, my question is - are sixty vitamins a day enough? I get it. I just want all women to have health throughout menopause regardless of their financial situation. I love how you call it "The seven Dwarfs of Menopause. Itchy, Bitchy, Sleepy, Sweaty, Bloated, Forgetful and All Dried Up."

I also read that the company Wyeth who makes Premarin, the HRT that is cruelly derived from pregnant horses, is trying to prevent women from having the choice of using compounded bio-identical hormones. Why? Because they are losing money since many women have stopped using Premarin and started using bio-identical hormones. It's mind boggling to know it is once again all about the profit with no regard to a woman's, and in this case a pregnant mare's, health or welfare.

I know we have to get back to my BHRT doctor and that urine test result, but yeah later. For now, I have a few more comments on pieces that I have read that have once again made me think: Oh, okaay!

217

Throughout my journey I have read that HRT's purpose is to rebalance our hormones. Oh really? Knowing what I know now about HRT I thought it was made to make me suffer more, shorten my life span, give me other health issues, take my money and to make me haemorrhage! Logically, HRT cannot rebalance our hormones. It is mass-produced and tossed on a shelf for profit only. It cannot be tailor made to suit a woman's individual needs. The only way to get safe, plant based, tailor made hormones back into your body is BHRT. This is my opinion but, as always, do what you feel is best for you.

There are also women out there who do not support other women through this phase of their lives. These women think that as menopause is a natural event, it should be "done" totally naturally, meaning with nothing, nada, zilch. Oh, okaay! These women also have the right to go through menopause in any way they choose, but they have no right to turn their noses up at, or try and put down, women who choose to find a therapy that helps alleviate their symptoms and suffering. Ladies, when your eyesight starts to go, are you going to do nothing about it because it is a natural part of life? Are you prepared to spend the rest of your lives bumping into things, being unable to read, and becoming a danger on our roads every time you drive? Yeah, think about it girls. I respect your decision to do menopause your way, but don't come near me or any other woman with those turned up noses and attitudes just because we choose to do it our way.

I read an article that stated that the health department wants women to take responsibility for their own health. Oh, okaay! They expect us to take responsibility for our own health but are not willing to educate us and provide us with the truth so that we *can* take responsibility for our own health! Are they now going to try and turn it around and make out it's our fault, because more women are standing up and saying they are not putting up with being guinea pigs anymore, are demanding more respect, and are demanding to be listened to?

I saw on TV a younger woman dealing with menopause who was saying many positive things about HRT, but she is only going to use it if her hot flushes get worse. Then I read that she works in the medical community and her husband is a doctor. Oh okaay! I hate to admit it but I had two thoughts: "How much are you and your doctor husband profiting in trying to make HRT sound so wonderful?" and "You are trying to encourage other women to use HRT but you are not using it yourself?" This is what I suggest to you sweetheart; put yourself on HRT and do a self-study for however long it takes, then get back to me and let me know how wonderful HRT is. You have a right to your opinion, but you have no right to sell HRT to following generations of women when you are not even using it yourself. I always thought it was disgusting that pharmaceutical companies are selling our health out for the almighty dollar. How much more horrible is it that another woman is selling us out for the $ sign too?

When I had that moment in the mental health unit, the team member asked me if I thought I was "reacting" to being menopausal? Oh okaay! I am all for food for thought, but I didn't even chew on this comment. So are you suggesting I was trying to take myself out of the whole menopausal scenario because I couldn't accept that I was menopausal? Like I was shaking my clenched fists up to heaven saying "WHY GOD WHY?" as I drop to my knees sobbing? Well, yeahnah. I was actually looking forward to having a menopausal party to celebrate her arrival. So no, I am not "reacting" to being menopausal, I am a menopausal woman losing major hormones that affect us in many, many ways, and I am still totally gob smacked by their attitude towards those of us going through this process.

Chapter 37

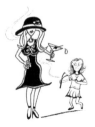

AND AN "I AM DISGUSTED"

While reading our local Sunday paper, (I am an avid reader of the horoscopes) I came to the Health Advice section. Here a woman in her 50s had written in asking for help with her "insufferable hot flushes." She knew they were caused by menopause, but just wanted to know how long they would last and also get some advice on how they could be managed.

The doctor's response started with information on hormone levels and how other factors can come into it if there is an abrupt or sudden drop in hormones, such as the surgical removal of the ovaries, chemotherapy and radiotherapy. The doctor also mentioned how men can even experience hot flushes and how their testosterone production is suppressed during times such as prostate cancer treatment. I am reading this and thinking, ok all good information but this woman has asked you for advice about her menopause symptoms. Did her concerns just get shoved aside, downplayed?

I think all information is fantastic, but I often see that when a woman asks for advice about menopause, the medical world seems to move on to other stuff, which gets away from the original question. Sometimes it veers off to talk about men's menopause as if to say, "What are you whinging for? Men might go through it as well." Or they suggest that a woman is only going to suffer greatly if other factors are involved. Did this just happen?

The doctor's next paragraph was a bit better. She spoke of how some women are only mildly affected, but also stated that some women suffer debilitating symptoms. She went on to say that symptoms are typically worse in the two years leading up to menopause. Huh? As we know now, there are three stages of menopause, so I assume she is talking about the two years before our periods stop. Where did she get those "facts" from?

Yes we know about the "roller coaster" effect before we officially stop our periods, but I personally only started to see physical symptoms in my body about six months before my period stopped, so from what I am reading she is saying the worst of it is in that time frame, that is, two years before menopause hits and our periods stop. Is she telling me that everything I have suffered since my periods ended is minor compared with what went before?

This doctor did go on and talk about herbal remedies such as dong guai, black cohosh, soy and others and how these might help. She also suggested minimizing stress, taking regular exercise, cold drinks, using a fan etc. She also told us to avoid hot foods, caffeine, alcohol and smoking. Ok all good, I guess. Hot flushes have not been a biggie for me, so for those dealing with hot flushes, it's up to you if you think this advice helps.

It also stated that symptoms tend to be more severe for those who are overweight, underweight or who have smoked. It made me think about my endocrinologist who said that originally they thought women who were thinner didn't suffer with hot flushes or night sweats as severely, but this thought was thrown out the window. So where did this doctor get her data from and how can she say that hot flushes can

221

be more severe if we are overweight or underweight? All I am thinking at the moment is, make up your bloody mind! Is it being overweight or underweight that causes severe hot flushes. The doctor then goes on to suggest if all else fails try HRT, but still does not mentioned BHRT as an option.

But it was the next bit that infuriated and disgusted me enough to shoot off an email to her. In the paragraph that says "How to Ease Symptoms," she said:

> Non-hormonal treatment options include some anti-depressants, an anticonvulsant medication and a medication usually used for controlling blood pressure.

She said that there could be some side effects. You think doc? I couldn't believe it! So off went the email saying:

> I am an avid reader of blah blah but I was disappointed and quite alarmed by the advice Dr blah gave in the Health Advice column dated blah blah. Firstly, why would you, Dr blah, suggest ant-depressants and anticonvulsant medications as a way of easing hot flushes? You did not even follow this through with any reasoning as to why you suggested these medications. I am absolutely gob smacked and quite frightened for the millions of menopausal women who may have read your column.

> Secondly why did you not give BHRT as another option for the menopausal woman to ponder? I understand that the normal response is that it is not scientifically proven, but the dangers that HRT pose to a woman have been proven and yet you still suggest it along side anti-depressants, anticonvulsant and another medicine, which you didn't even bother to name, that controls blood pressure!

> In your first paragraph you made it sound as if women will only suffer greatly through menopause if other factors come into play and I also understand that some men may have a form of menopause as well, but every woman in the world in every generation will deal with menopause, so why the flippant attitude towards the fact that many healthy women

with all their bits intact still have a debilitating journey through menopause?

I also understand that a change in lifestyle is always great at any time in our lives, but there are many women who have never smoked or even tasted alcohol who suffer greatly with hot flushes. I also know women who do smoke and drink alcohol who do not suffer with hot flushes or night sweats but deal with other symptoms. Can you please explain that to me?

As a menopausal woman who has being dealing with it since 2010 and who now is living with another illness due to menopause, it is time for doctors to be made more accountable for the advice they may see fit to give the menopausal woman. We are in the 21st Century not the 1800s where the menopausal woman was treated physically, mentally and emotionally in a way that is heart breaking.

To end I must also say I had quite a few calls from friends after reading your column who were just as disgusted with your advice to the woman who was needing help with her hot flushes.

So there you go. I am just so disgusted with some of the advice that comes from the so-called experts. It worries me. Not only did an article once again divert from and down play a woman's suffering by taking the focus off the main question for a while, and not only are all the options for the menopausal woman still not being put out into the main stream, but an expert is advising the use of anti-depressants, anticonvulsant and other medication to ease hot flushes? I didn't think the battle for the rights and the wellbeing of menopausal women could get any bigger, well it just did! I will wait and see if I get a response and if and when I do, as usual, I will let you know—hopefully in the future.

Chapter 38

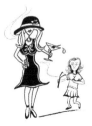

BACTERIA IN THE GUT

Ok I guess it's time to find out what is happening with my urine test. Apparently the urine test results show that I have a heap of bad bacteria in my gut. The highest reading or level for these buggers hanging around in your gut is four. My results were sitting at three and a half. I had noticed, putting my bloating and my fatty liver to the side, that in the last week or two I was feeling a little nauseated but nothing too bad. I had also noticed that I was giving my stomach a bit of a rub because of it, but that was it.

I asked my doctor if I should have noticed something if the bad bacterial count was this high. He said that it could have been sitting around ready to happen for a few years. My first thought was Ms Menopause has been hanging around for years. This has to connect to her somehow. I also thought, so much for my cast iron stomach, but maybe it is *because* of my cast iron stomach that I haven't suffered the normal side affects I would have expected.

I had to do a gut cleansing that involved a special diet, and then build up to eighteen tablets a day, oh, that would make it twenty tablets a day if you include my steroids. I would also have to go off the daily antibiotic that the allergist started me on, and which I have been on for over two months now. This gut programme was to continue for ten to fourteen days, then we would work on building up the good bacteria in my stomach again.

I walked out of there knowing I had told my BHRT doctor that I would go off the antibiotics so I could do this. I also walked out of there with scripts for these three tablets I would need to take. All I could think of was "Twenty tablets? A day?" Geez, I now felt like that actress in one of those midday shows that sounds like "As the Stomach Churns." I just need a glass of vodka to down them all with. Twelve of these eighteen tablets were all-natural, so that made me feel a bit better.

I knew also that I had to have real faith in someone in the medical community and decided the BHRT doctor was it. I did ask the universe to help me make the right decision. I also did some heavy duty praying to the universe to keep me safe if I did have a reaction. I then brought all my tablets home and started the Gut Restoration process. The plan was to build up to two of these three tablets, three times a day. Because of my allergies and my immune system, he advised me to build up slowly, and if there wasn't a problem to continue to build up to the eighteen a day.

It took three days to get to three tablets. For the next two days I was able to build up to nine tablets a day. I was taking one of the three tablets, three times a day. I was a little puffy and a little redness was becoming visible. I was ok and not getting worse, but I was keeping a good eye on it. In the next few days I had to have a day off them altogether as I woke up quite puffy, and the redness was turning into a bit of a rash. I was able to get back on one of the three tablets daily and I sat semi comfortable on those three until it was time to stop.

So now I just had to wait, do another urine test and see if the bad bacteria count was lower and go from there. I have noticed I am not rubbing my gut anymore and my stomach doesn't seem to be as bloated; well my BHRT doctor did say it would also help with my fatty liver.

When I had gone to the chemist to get the scripts filled for the tablets, I had a chat to the young pharmacist there. He explained to me that the long-term use of steroids could cause these infestations of bacteria. He did explain it in full but I was quite tired and I zoned out a bit. When I came home and read up on the information sheet it also stated that antibiotic therapy could cause it. Bingo! I knew this all had to tie in with Ms Menopause. I am only on steroids and long-term antibiotics because of her. Yeah you are good Ms Menopause, sneaky, cunning, but very clever.

I just want to have a quick chat to my cast iron stomach. "Don't worry girl, we will get through this. One day you and I will be sitting together again eating and drinking whatever we want, just like the good old days. You have done me proud throughout all these years, just hang in there. Yeah and I agree that *she* is a bitch, but anger won't do you any good, just try and relax and get better."

I have been on my new finely tuned BHRT for five weeks and I will tell you not one drop of blood have I had to sacrifice while on this, unlike HRT which nearly drained me of all the blood in my body! I am due to do another "saliva spit thing" as I did on St Valentine's Day and get it tested to see how my new progesterone levels are. Both this result and the gut restoration results will be known in about a week when I see my BHRT doctor again.

I will say that in just under three weeks of being on my BHRT, I noticed my energy levels were a little higher and even loved ones had noticed. I still drag the chain with my health and yes, I have to be aware that the steroids mask my ills as well, but this wee bit of extra energy just felt different. It felt like it wasn't coming from the steroids, as they can do that at times. This energy came before I started the gut restoration thing, which has dragged me back a bit, but it was too important not to do that. Yeah, this energy felt like *me*.

I have had a couple of bigger off-days with my skin and energy caused by the gut restoration, but as I said, I have put faith in my BHRT doctor and I really need my cast iron stomach to be strong and healthy when, god willing, the BHRT does it's thing long term, and we are better and have energy, and are able to have a nice lunch with a lovely cold chardy without puffing up and getting inflamed, and without my skin turning red and getting a rash, and without me trying to take myself out due to the menopause induced depression.

Not only did this energy feel like me, I also felt deep down in my soul a little stirring of happiness. Maybe putting the wee bit of energy and the little stirring of happiness together is building up my health and wellbeing again. I know I have a long way to go with my health, but I have to put it all into perspective. Looking back over this long journey of trying to get my health back and actually making it into old age healthy, happy and able, well a few bigger "off" days now is still better than where I have been.

I really have to make note that on the 29th of October 2013 I wrote down that it was a good day. My soul felt it was waking up but I have learnt not get too excited at times as the next day I can crash and burn again. But honestly, this is the first time I have felt stirrings of me again throughout this whole struggle. We shall wait and see.

Chapter 39

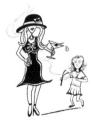

THE LOGIC OF MS MENOPAUSE

Until the secrecy and invisible blanket are lifted around menopause, and women are told the truth and are educated so that they can take control of their own health, there is no logic to Ms Menopause. We cannot work out the logic without the facts.

I am only now, on this journey, taking control of my own health and gaining more knowledge about Ms Menopause, but if I had known earlier what I know now, I may not have had to live on steroids, antibiotics and all the rest.

These are the facts I have found through my research about our bodies and how they are affected:

Oestrogen - sex hormone: This is made in the adrenal glands, ovaries and fatty tissue. It assists with the growth of the uterus lining in the beginning of our period cycle. It maintains bone strength by working with calcium, vitamin D and other minerals to prevent bone loss. So in menopause this is why we lose bone density. It's caused by the loss of estrogen.

Progesterone: This is produced in the ovaries and adrenal tissue. It prepares the uterus for the egg to be planted. Apparently progesterone production starts to decrease in women in their forties and throughout menopause. Low levels can cause irritability, mood swings, weight gain, depression, pain and osteoporosis. Throughout menopause progesterone goes all the way down to nada. Estrogen also goes down but we keep approximately forty percent of it, hence the estrogen dominance and the above menopausal symptoms.

Testosterone: I really haven't mentioned much about this, but it is produced in small amounts in women. It is made by steroid hormones that are produced by the adrenal glands. Yep, we keep coming back to those two little suckers, the adrenal glands! It increases a woman's energy levels and libido and strengthens bones and muscles.

Adrenal Glands: Yeah I am going to add these in here. I've already talked about their role. These little suckers are really important through life but more so when a woman is dealing with Ms Menopause.

Above is a simple breakdown of their functions, but I felt it was enough to understand their workings, why make it more complicated than is needed. I will leave that up to the medical community. Yes, did you catch the sarcasm?

I have always found that finding the logic helps, so I will give you some "logics" that I have found:

During menopause our ovaries stop producing most of our estrogen and all of our progesterone, and due to the body's hormones and glands relying on each other, it is logical that with these losses, other "side dish" symptoms may appear. So the pain you are feeling in one part of your body can be caused by problems in another part of your body. Here are some examples:

- Lower back pain could be due to chronic adrenal stress. It leads to weakness in the muscles that support the pelvis. Pain may be due to instability in your pelvis, but the core of this problem comes from adrenal gland exhaustion.
- Loss of oestrogen affects our brain and lowers serotonin levels. This is considered to be our "happy" hormone. It affects our overall sense of well-being. It is logical that we may experience menopause-induced depression.
- The adrenal glands, if healthy, kick in and produce estrogen to help women through menopause. It is logical that if the adrenal glands are exhausted or fatigued, a woman's suffering through menopause will be greater.
- I also now see the logic in estrogen dominance. We are going to have estrogen dominance if we keep using HRT as it has more estrogen in it. What we need is progesterone. Even if HRT is not being used due to the uneven drops of these two hormones, we still will get estrogen dominance naturally.

So looking at these few "logics", the actual process of menopause is very simple. Hear that Ms Menopause? You yourself are not that big at all. You are only getting away with so much because, when it comes to you, the medical community in this 21st century still has the mentality of the medical community of the 1800s. So a natural part of a woman's life is being allowed to branch out into bigger and much scarier health issues which we billions of "ovary keepers" know now should not be happening. Yeah I still reckon there is a lot of power in our ovaries.

Oh, and a word on insulin. It's a hormone produced by the pancreas. It is also a protein made up of fifty-one amino acids. Now I shall list these in detail. Yeahnah! Just joking! If you really want to get to know the fifty-one amino acids, you are on your own. Something I have been stunned by throughout this journey with Ms Menopause are the things I didn't know and really didn't have any interest in concerning my body, including these facts on insulin. Insulin, for some reason, has amused me. I went from thinking it comes from a syringe in liquid form for those who need it, to knowing it is actually a hormone in our body. I am sure those of you who are insulin dependent and have to have daily blood pricks and injections are not amused by my amusement. No disrespect is intended. I am just in awe of how clever our bodies are and I'm in awe of how every bit of us, if not functioning properly, can cause such a huge ripple effect throughout the rest of our body.

I am starting to get the same amusement from the gall bladder. Have you ever heard someone say, "The gall of that person?" It means to be bold and not show respect for another. I think I might have to investigate the gall bladder, I am hoping the gall bladder hasn't got the gall to do me any more damage whilst I am dealing with Ms Menopause! I remember listing it as a symptom. I will let you know, "I'll Be Back."

I'm back! The gallbladder sits under the liver. It serves as a reservoir until the bile is needed in the small intestine to digest fats. This need is signalled by a hormone called cholecystokinin, this hormone then makes the gallbladder contract and deliver bile into the intestine. Excess estrogen from HRT appears to increase cholesterol levels in bile and decreases the movement of the gallbladder, which can lead to gallstones. Gallstones happen when the bile isn't released as it should and it builds up into a stone of bile, yuk!

Oestrogen is broken down in the liver. During the early stage of menopause the estrogen levels can be higher at times, remember the roller coaster effect? This then makes the liver work harder which produces more bile, which in turn puts stress on the gallbladder. This is why we menopausal women are at higher risk of getting gallbladder stones than the general population.

Studies have shown that HRT doubles or even triples the risk of gallstones, hospitalization for gall bladder disease or gallbladder surgery. Symptoms of having gallstones are pain in the stomach area, or in the upper right part of your belly under the ribs. It can cause vomiting, and from what I have researched the pain is pretty damn bad. Our body weight change is the most common factor for the gall bladder problems. This is skimming over the symptoms, and as usual, with any change or pain in your body, consult your doctor and make them listen to you.

So that is gallstone's story. I am sure none of us were surprised to see that the gall bladder did have the gall to also give us a hard time through menopause. So it is a sack full of bile. Vile! You are never too old to learn something new.

Ok, now back to my BHRT doc for results. You know we are now in December 2013 and Christmas is just on the horizon. I want to get these results from my BHRT doctor then hopefully put it all away until next year. Anyhoo we couldn't get a result from the gut restoration plan as my body wouldn't allow me to be on all the tablets I needed. My BHRT doctor thought it wasn't worth testing my urine as I have to pay to get this special test done, so we are looking into that again next year, but as I mentioned, my gut does feel better. The results of the saliva test showed that I had a bit too much progesterone in my body and my BHRT doctor asked how I was travelling since I went down in the amount of progesterone I was using. Huh?

Apparently he had requested that I be called a week ago to advise me of this. Well, no call came through with that information so we just got it sorted while I was there. I had been having quite severe headaches in the last couple of weeks and spoke to my BHRT doc about these. The headaches were quite harsh and really hurt. I was actually getting a bit concerned but knew I would get checked if they continued. He said it could be due to coming down in steroids; he then said that it could be due to having too much BHRT in my body.

My BHRT doctor also wants to test me for Addison's disease because of the discolouring of my skin from my wrist to my elbow. Yes, my skin is now discoloured. If I bumped my skin in this area I would bleed. Another doctor had originally told me that the discolouration of my skin was caused by iron left under my skin due to the bleeding. My doctor first had to find out how to be tested for Addison's disease, so again I am happy to hang it all up until next year.

Before walking out I did check with reception as to what phone number they had in my records. They told me, but I assumed it was an old one, which I really didn't comprehend as I had to fill out a new patient's sheet when I first saw my BHRT doc, and I know I would have put my current number on. Anyway we just updated my records. When I reached home I remembered I had forgotten to book an appointment for the daughter to see my BHRT doctor so just rang them. This now leads me into all that came next. When I rang them and told them who I was and that I was booking an appointment for my daughter I was asked, "Which Jenni Townsend are you?" All I could come back with was, "You are joking aren't you, there are two of me there as well?" I then had to go on and explain my reaction. This is a different medical centre and has nothing to do with my new allergist who is seeing two of me, that is two Jenni Townsend's, as well.

I hadn't been asked that before so it got me thinking that this other Jenni Townsend must have started seeing my doc after me. The appointment was made for a week later. The daughter asked if I would go with her and as we were guided into his room the daughter had forgotten her juice in the waiting room and dashed out to grab it. While we had a moment, this happened:

BHRT Doc: So how is your rash going?

Me: [Knowing my skin was sort of holding] "You mean this?" [pointing to my discolouration]

BHRT Doc: No, when you rang the other day to say you were having a reaction to…

Well he said the name of a medication I knew I wasn't using. Right there and then the light bulb switched on for both of us at the same time.

BHRT Doc: Oh no, no that's not you.

Me: [The daughter walks back in to see me putting my hand up in a STOP fashion towards the BHRT doctor and saying] "Please do not get me mixed up with the other Jenni Townsend, this has already happened to me with my new allergist!

Yep! What can I say? Was that Jenni Townsend's phone number instead of mine? Maybe not because I haven't had to field any calls for her! So, now there are THREE OF US? Oh dear I can hear some of you thinking, I reckon one of me is enough, but three? I started to think that they are following me around, but they could be thinking I am the stalker! I wonder if they are experiencing all the stuff I have had to deal with as well? It's mind blowing that the obstacles and hurdles just continue to come at me. I know this was only minor, but this is when I decided I was going to add in the obstacles section but am choosing to call it, with tongue in cheek, I think....

Chapter 40

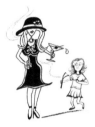

THE MENOPAUSE CONSPIRACY

I really chewed over whether to put all the following in but decided to as all these obstacles have only happened since Ms Menopause arrived. Ok, it is logical to say that if I had had the truth and education at the beginning of this journey I wouldn't have dealt with any of the following, but surely the following is not the norm. Could it also be said that most of the following is due to the fact that menopause is not taken seriously in mainstream society, and that the medical community and different departments have decided to hide and dismiss the truth and seriousness of menopause?

So here is a list of all the obstacles I have had to face since *she* turned up:

We all know about Centrelink where I was put on Newstart Allowance and had that bloody employment agency hounding me, OBSTACLE 1.

Then I was advised I owed them money even though I had a doctor's certificate covering me for that time period, OBSTACLE 2.

The second attempt with Centrelink made it quite obvious by the voice on the other end of the phone that no one knows where to "put" the menopausal woman who is suffering, OBSTACLE 3.

After a bit of time had passed since I had left work, I realized that this was not just going to take a month to get better so I rang my superannuation company to ask if I was covered by a certain payment. I was told no. OBSTACLE 4.

(I know I have to put my hand up for some of the fault here. Yeah I get a yearly superannuation statement but never looked into what it covered. It was always a quick look and a, "That will be a nice amount when I retire at seventy," but that was it. I then had to utilize my saved superannuation, which required their doctor's certificates needing to be filled out by my doctor and my first allergist, which were done and submitted to get my super released.)

As stated by the young bloke who was handling this for me, the release of my funds was taking longer than normal, OBSTACLE 5.

Throughout the to and fro contact with my super company, I was accidently transferred to a different department who advised me that I did indeed have cover for that certain payment, and that the policy was being paid through my superannuation. So now funds were kept in my super account to keep paying this policy so that I could claim for the other payment. When it came to my super funds being released, they apparently couldn't transfer my money straight into my account even though there had never been a problem with transferring in and out of my account in the last nineteen years. OBSTACLE 6.

This then meant a cheque had to be drawn, sent off for authorization, received in the mail, and clearance time put on it, which caused a longer time that my funds were held up, OBSTACLE 7.

Ok that was finally sorted and new paperwork was sent to me to be filled out to get the other payment. Just dealing with the above was so stressful for me I knew I wouldn't be able, health wise, to deal with the next stage of it on my own, so I spoke to a lawyer who I have known since my daughter was three. He agreed to take it on for me and I would pay him when this next lot of "pocket money" came in.

This new paperwork required another certificate needing to be filled out by my doctor, which was also an employment statement to be filled out by my previous employer. I thought I could handle the employment statement myself, but after sending three emails to the human resources team in Sydney requesting the address I needed to send this paperwork to, I was getting no replies. I had even cc'd one of my emails to the human resources manager, OBSTACLE 8.

I ended up getting a reply, but it was just a statement saying that I had worked there and not what I had requested, OBSTACLE 9.

My lawyer took this on for me as I couldn't handle the stress involved. After he requested the required information, the form was filled out and received in seven days. The human resources manager was even having contact with my lawyer. Go figure eh! The human resources manager said that the team member must have misunderstood what I was requesting. Oh really? So she misunderstood: COULD YOU PLEASE ADVISE WHAT ADDRESS I NEED TO SEND THIS PAPERWORK TO SO THAT IT CAN BE FILLED OUT. Oh and let's not forget she "misunderstood" it three times. Ok rightio! A big whatever back at you! I also asked my lawyer why the insurance company now requires more doctors' certificates to be completed? He said that they will say that we are now dealing with a different section.

All paperwork initially requested by the insurance company has finally been submitted. My lawyer then received an email requesting that I was to obtain all clinical records not only from my doctor, but now also from my first allergist. This gets OBSTACLE 10 due to more time being wasted, whereas if we had known all this was needed initially, it would have all been sent with the original claim. My very professional lawyer swung an email back to them stating that they were to do this, which they did. This is where the first allergist was able to affect my finances. I need to give the first allergist more paper space, and you too will feel you have just walked into the "Twilight Zone."

Ok, all records received by the insurance company from my doctor, goody! The insurance company then rang the first allergist practice where I had last seen him in 2012. The insurance company was then told by his receptionist that I had not seen him there in 2012, OBSTACLE 11.

My lawyer asked me to confirm the details that had been sent to the insurance company and I did this. Now the insurance company is requesting the first allergist to also fill out their doctor's certificate. I know it sounds like splitting hairs but the insurance company certificate needs more detail, and fair enough I initially thought.

Even though this first allergist had filled out a similar form of certificate previously, trying to get him to fill out this next form, and just getting his report on me through the years, was like pulling teeth! Why is this? And not just with him, why is it so hard to get reports released once you have seen a doctor or specialist? It makes me feel they need to rub stuff out before it gets released. It's easy, I come to see you, you record what is wrong with me, you try and fix me, you get paid big money, but to get a copy of this in report form is like trying to get blood from a rock! Yeah I just don't get it.

My doctor rang the first allergist's practice where I had seen him in 2011 and was told by his receptionist that the last time I had seen the first allergist there was 2008! Yep! OBSTACLE 12.

My doctor then told her that he wanted to speak to the first allergist in regard to filling out this insurance certificate that was needed. She told him, "He doesn't do that," meaning, he doesn't fill out forms. OBSTACLE 13.

So! Let's have a think about all this before I continue. Both the insurance company and my own doctor have now been told by two different receptionists at the two different practices that I have not seen this first allergist since 2008 or even at all.

I know all this sounds very unemotional, but I have to try and divorce myself from it emotionally as I type. I can assure you that there was a lot of emotion and distress involved when it was actually happening. I am just finding with this "Menopause Conspiracy" I need to try not to relive all that emotion again as it is just too damn hard, and to be honest it ain't good for my health!

Ok, so I have receipts of payment for the desensitisation injections the first allergist organized in 2011and 2012. There is more that can be traced back to these two appointments, but now I feel I have to prove I saw him! OBSTACLE 14.

What a load of crap! Luckily the injections, once mixed, were sent to my doctor's practice to be given by his nurses. Imagine if the first allergist had done them, would he say that they were never done? Who knows? I also say thank goodness for Medicare on-line as it shows that the first allergist bulked billed me for the visits in 2011 and 2012. I was quite surprised to see these two bulk bills on my statement as I thought my payment covered all, but I was also elated to see them too!

Moving on, it took a phone call from my lawyer to get this first allergist's report sent to them. When it finally came through it was just his written material about me over the years I had been seeing him, but when my lawyer sent it to me to ensure all was in order before it was sent to the insurance company, it was full of contradictions and false statements, OBSTACLE 15.

I was absolutely gobsmacked. It took me a whole weekend to just digest it all then I sent a letter off to my lawyer responding to his material paragraph by paragraph. The best part of it all though was his little add-in at the bottom stating that he didn't recall ever filling out a form for me in regard to my superannuation and that it must have been another allergist or dermatologist, OBSTACLE 16.

So he is stating that he didn't fill out the first form. Ok we have a copy of the form filled out in his hand writing, with the original form sent off to the super company in 2012 to get my super funds released, which they were, and he is saying he never filled this form out. Oh really?

Now just to fill you in, my claim with the insurance company was submitted in March 2013, this crock of crap was received by the first allergist in May 2013, so two months, so far, have been wasted stuffing around with this twit. Oh yeah and a note to the first allergist: You said it may have been another medical person who filled the form out for me, well I may be unwell and my clarity and concentration may be out at times, but I am an intelligent woman. I would have been fully aware if I was seeing another allergist or dermatologist at that time! I guess the blessing in disguise was that all this pushed me into actually organizing another allergist.

Trying to get the first allergist to fill out the certificate went on for a little while longer but in the end his paperwork regarding me had to be sent "as is" to the insurance company. The end result was that the first allergist refused to fill out another report, OBSTACLE 17.

And he was removed from my claim with the insurance company. So time wasted over this bloke turned into a good four months or more, OBSTACLE 18.

I always thought it was a medical specialists legal obligation to fill out forms as requested for their patients when needed. Nobody has asked him to do anything except tell it as it is. No one has his arm twisted behind his back telling him to write untruths. He has just been asked to do his bloody job! However I do now understand the need for them to perhaps "rub out and try again" when requesting a copy of a report. This just proves that they could be writing anything about you, but the bottom line is, people, those reports are about me, so why all the hardship involved in getting a copy of it? Interestingly enough though, in the first allergist's material he wrote in detail about my two appointments with him in 2011 and 2012 and then he wrote "One contributing factor is considered to be menopause." Phew! Thank god he mentioned this, for a moment I was sure I didn't see him in 2011 and 2012 and that I wasn't even dealing with menopause! Ha ha he he chuckle chuckle. As if!

So now the first allergist has been put out to pasture regarding my claim, actually I think he should be put out to pasture literally. This first allergist, this professor who has had a very long career as a doctor of this and a fellow of that and a member of this and that, and who was also listed in "Who's Who in Australia" at one time, really concerns me. Who in the medical world is watching these doctors and specialists ensuring they are still able to practice in an ethical and safe way in regard to their patients? Yeah it concerns me greatly that he is still out there practicing and I believe due to this first allergist's flippant attitude to menopause, he has put my chance of survival back a year or two.

Moving on to my new allergist, it took a good seven weeks to get his report, after numerous requests, so that it could be sent to the insurance company, OBSTACLE 19.

We all know what went down when I finally did have it in hand, yes, the wrong Jenni Townsend's personal details were on my report. OBSTACLE 20.

Before I continue I am going to make the Medical World's flippant attitude towards the menopausal woman OBSTACLE 21.

Their flippant attitude towards menopause itself is OBSTACLE 22.

The Medical World saying that the suffering many women may experience through menopause is just a part of getting old, OBSTACLE 23.

For downplaying my debilitating journey through it, OBSTACLE 24.

For that third "me" whom I have been mixed up with down at my BHRT doctor's medical centre, OBSTACLE 25.

She must be following me because I was seeing him first. Hmm. Maybe I am just getting a wee paranoid. Oh! I wonder why!

The new allergist's report was sent into the insurance company on October 21st 2013. I was finally starting to feel we were in the home stretch of all this mess. I actually thought all the obstacles were behind me. I know I am very fortunate that my lawyer and his team have taken this on for me, but the stress and emotions I still had to invest in all of this was just too much. All this crap was going on around me when I just needed to try and focus on my health. But no, it wasn't over yet, and the following was when I totally got over it all. Only now? I can hear some of you thinking. Yeah I know. Looking back on it though, my personal opinion in regard to the first allergist is that after a long career I don't think he is capable of practicing safely due to his age. I don't think what went down with him was deliberate sabotage against me. Who in their right mind would say I didn't see him in 2011 and 2012 then write about both these appointments he had with me? Who in their right mind would say he didn't fill out that first doctor's certificate in 2012 when we have the proof to say, "Ummm yeah ya did buster."

What came next though made me realize that perhaps "fair play" was not at hand in regard to the insurance company, and I thank God my lawyer was involved as I was sitting slumped in the backseat as he dealt head on with this next Goliath.

And so for OBSTACLE 26. Seven months have now been wasted between the first allergist and the time it took to get the second allergist's report submitted to the insurance company. Ok so the new allergist's report went through in October 2013. I understand things take time, but three weeks had passed with no word about my claim. My lawyer has been wonderful, and as I am not his only client I don't expect him to be giving me daily updates. I appreciate the fact that he knows I am struggling with my health and need to concentrate on that, but to be able to do this I need my pocket money. So after this time lapsed I sent an email off to him asking if there had been any communication regarding my claim. He advised me that they had already started to chase up my claim with no word as yet, but yes, they were keeping on top of it.

A few days later an email came through from my lawyer stating that the insurance company had made, and were paying for, an appointment for me to see a dermatologist. Ok, I didn't have a problem with this but I did have a problem with the fact that they expected me to wait another five weeks until December 12th before I saw this dermatologist so, OBSTACLE 27.

It is now over seven weeks that my claim will just sit dormant since October, OBSTACLE 28.

I did shoot back an email to my lawyer asking if this appointment could possibly be brought forward.

I learnt here that there is a cycle which goes like this: I communicate with my lawyer and his team. My lawyer deals with my superannuation company who then deals with the insurance company. I received a call from my lawyer a week later saying that they had requested for this appointment to be brought forward and that they would stay on the case, but the superannuation company, they say, told my lawyer that they were not getting a response from the insurance company, OBSTACLE 29.

On the 4th of December we were advised that no, the set date could not be brought forward, OBSTACLE 30.

All I could say to my lawyer is, "Ok then, but that's bad form." Why bad form? Well this is why: once this appointment was set for me it was made very clear that I had to confirm my attendance by the 5th December. If I had said, "No I am not going," or cancelled after the 5th of December, I would have to pay the insurance company $1000. Hmmm, and we all know how that would have been paid... with buttons! I don't think the insurance company even tried to change the date. I don't believe it was just coincidence that they only advised us of this on the 4th of December, one day before I had to confirm. It could be said that they tried their damned hardest to get it changed right up to the confirmation date, but nah. This insurance company wasn't even responding to emails sent to them from the superannuation company, or so they say. And this insurance company had just under four weeks to either get it changed or to advise us earlier. I also get that some specialists have a waiting period because they're popular, but all the insurance company was asked to do was make a phone call, see if my appointment could be booked earlier and that was it, so even if December 12th was the only appointment left with this dermatologist, I would have thought they had ample time to advise us, but no, they didn't even bother to try and get the date changed. This was my first taste of seeing that fair play is not how they operate, OBSTACLE 31.

It made me realize that there is not much care or concern from the superannuation company and as for the insurance company, what came next was unacceptable and just confirmed what I had been thinking about my "not playing fair" conspiracy. There doesn't seem to be any form of urgency from anyone except me. I know there are rules and regulations to follow, but maybe they are all waiting for me to say, "Ok you got me, I am just pretending to be this sick. Oh well gave that my best shot, oh and menopause doesn't even exist," and head back into life. Perhaps they could even be waiting for me to "croak" so that they don't have to pay me what I am entitled to. I dunno!

Before we get into the next obstacle let's chat about that $1000 bucks for a moment. So, if I didn't want to go for no good reason, or if I cancel now that I have confirmed my attendance, I then have to pay the insurance company $1000 bucks. Wow. This dermatologist must have some magic up his sleeve to be able to charge that much. Maybe he can "lay hands" on me and cure my menopause, stop my immune system from attacking itself and give me back those pert young breasts I once had. I reckon for that cost I should be in for a back massage and able to bring him home to do a few hours of housework, food shopping, cooking and wash the exterior of our house.

I assume that this is his fee as he is only a ten-minute drive away from home and there is no travelling or accommodation costs needed to be paid by the insurance company. If it's not the fee he charges then the insurance company is making money off me. Huh? I get sick and have to pay the insurance company $1000 bucks? Double huh! What a little money-spinner that is. Imagine if he saw three of me and we all know that could be a possibility. Yeah, I am definitely starting to feel that I would like to know what the dermatologist's relationship with the insurance company is. Paying a specialist for their "expert" opinion is sure as hell cheaper than paying me my pocket money, even if this dermatologist does end up seeing the three of us. I will be spewing if I ever find out that either of the other two "me's" were also seeing him and got in to see him earlier than me. Anyhooo moving on.

It still takes all my might to get to my appointments but at least, well I thought, once I see this dermatologist it is done. All finished just before Christmas 2013, and all my tests my BHRT doctor want to do are hung up until next year, what the insurance company has requested of me is done and dusted, I don't see my new allergist until late January 2014 and I saw my own doctor earlier in December before he headed off for his holiday. As usual I am tired and exhausted. I know I haven't been able to work now for seventeen months but to have a break away from it all with no appointments to attend for a little while, well that felt like a holiday to me.

I used to have a great work ethic in my place of employment and was happy to work hard for my dollars, but since the knock on my door from Ms Menopause I don't think I have had to work as hard before in my entire life as I have had to for my health. To just continue to "be" and maintain some form of health has been the hardest, most exhausting, challenging, obstacle-filled, scariest and expensive position I have ever been in. Oh, and let's not forget, the pay is damn lousy too!

I rocked up for this appointment knowing I was a little early. I walked through the main doors straight into the front reception area then stated who I was, who I was to see and at what time.

Girl: Yes we do have a Dr blah blah here but he is not here now.

Me: But I have an appointment booked with him today.

Girl: [Pointing me through to another receptionist's desk] You might be best to see them and they may be able to sort it out for you.

(Now you would think something would be registering with me by now, but no, all the obstacles are behind me now, aren't they? I am just at the wrong reception area. Again I state who I am blah blah blah.)

New Girl: [Looking at me quite blankly] Did you mean you are to see Dr blah blah?

Me: No I am to see Dr blah blah as per instructed by the insurance company.

You know there was NO appointment on their computer for me to see this dermatologist on this day the 12th of December 2013. OBSTACLE 32.

And that explained their blank looks when I turned up as they were not expecting me. I told them I was heading out for a minute to ring my lawyer. I knew I was at the right place on the right day at the right time but still felt the need to confirm it with my lawyer. Once this was done I went back in. I'd say from what happened next the two receptionists did a bit of "looking into it" whilst I was out talking to my lawyer.

New Girl: What is your date of birth?

Me: Blah blah blah

New Girl: Ok, now there was an appointment made for you on the 9th of December, but it was cancelled. OBSTACLE 33.

Me: Oh ok, so was this appointment cancelled due to me not turning up for it as I was not aware of it?

New Girl: No the insurance company had cancelled it previously. OBSTACLE 34.

Me: Rightio then, thanks.

I then went out to call my lawyer again but due to all the emotions I was feeling, as soon as I heard his voice I couldn't get it out as I was sobbing so bloody hard. I told him, as best as I could, that I would send an email to him detailing it all as soon as I got home. I then went back to my car and called a loved one but that was futile in itself as I still continued to sob. After that call I just sat in the car to dry off a bit as I had decided to go back in and see if I could get that 9th of December cancelled appointment printed out. The girl advised me that it would be best if my lawyer rang them in the morning.

Only now, and not even by the first receptionist at the main reception area, was I advised of this:

New Girl: Oh and the doctor's surname you said is actually his middle name, his surname is actually blaaaah. I hope that is clearer now for you. OBSTACLE 35.

Me: Yep as clear as mud.

I did thank them both for letting me know. I sat in my car for a moment trying to wrap my head around it all then drove home.

What the hell just happened? Not only is there not an appointment made for me but the insurance company couldn't even give me this dermatologist's correct full name! I am constantly feeling like the walking dead and I had to walk into that? I really don't understand all the obstacles I have had to deal with throughout this journey. I do though, understand I am up against it most times as soon as I mention the word menopause, but so many obstacles and they aren't finished yet? I've just got to keep the faith and believe that all that is happening is for a reason and is meant to be and that up the track, once all of this is said and done, I will have that moment of, "Ahhh! Now I understand why that all had to happen."

I have to admit it just feels like too much at times. I know my lawyer is at the helm, but the stress I still have to deal with seems too big and overwhelming for me at times. Interestingly enough, when I was sobbing down the phone to my lawyer, I got a sense of the old, independent, strong me, the one that was around before Ms Menopause knocked. Now I want to talk about her for a moment, separated from me. It felt like this "me" had her back leaning up against a wall with arms crossed and her head cocked to one side watching all this go down. I can tell you that she was not impressed at all with what she was seeing and hearing.

Oh my god, maybe this obstacle did crack me. I am sobbing heavily down the phone into my lawyer's ear, but I am still getting a sense of the strong independent woman I use to be? It doesn't make sense! But yes, it does. When I got home and thought about it, I realised that the independent, strong woman I used to be was not impressed that I was put in a position by the insurance company that made me sob down the phone into the ear of a man that I have no emotional attachment to whatsoever. Don't get me wrong, I believe crying is good for you at times and have cried in the ear of some before, and to be honest my loved ones have never seen me cry as much before Ms Menopause arrived, but this was different.

This wasn't Ms Menopauses doing, although it did stem from her. This happened purely because of the actions of the superannuation and insurance companies. I was now sobbing in the ear of this lawyer who I had respected for a very long time? My lawyer didn't mind and was very compassionate, but I can tell you I minded! Right there and then we, oh I mean we girls, "me, myself and I," decided we didn't like the feel of what had just gone down and that enough was enough. Fair play from the insurance company was very obviously and definitely off the table now. You know I am all for mistakes. We are all human and we all make our own mistakes throughout our lives, I understand stuff happens, but my senses are telling me that this wasn't just human error.

Before I continue, I really hope you are all on the edge of your seats wondering, "What happens next?" I am not intentionally trying to bore you with this, but I really feel that it is all too important to leave out. Is this the norm for everyone who gets ill and has to leave their workplace, or am I copping it more because the word menopause is involved? In the dealings I have had with many since Ms M rocked up, I really believe I am being treated differently because I dare to stand up, even if it was only a whisper at times, to the many offhand attitudes that are out there towards menopause.

Would I have been more silent if I had known what was ahead of me? Ha ha he he chuckle chuckle, no way! Yes it has been a hard slog health-wise, stress-wise, financially-wise, plus physically, emotionally and mentally. Yes the ripple effect it has all had on my loved ones is heartbreaking. Yes I have had to be in the firing line of many a comment that could deem me to be a moron and the lack of respect for the menopause woman is there too, but I yam what I yam today due to Ms Menopause and nothing is going to change that. Why would I have any sense of needing to hide it? I know who I was before Ms Menopause knocked and I know who I am not anymore since her arrival.

I have always ensured though, when it all started to look like Ms Menopause was not involved at all, that my lawyer also kept Ms Menopause at the top of the list. Regardless of what the end result of all this is for me, I have stood my ground in making sure that all that I have battled against and all my lawyer is battling against, is that Ms Menopause is known as the culprit who started it all.

At home after that debacle with the dermatologist, once I had the energy, I sent an email off to my lawyer walking him through all that I had walked into. Things happened pretty fast. My lawyer was on the phone to the insurance company first thing the next morning with a "please explain" attitude, and also letting them know that what had happened was completely unacceptable.

What came next though moves us away from the "Twilight Zone" and straight into, as far as I am concerned, the "Big Black Hole of Bullshit Zone". Definition of Bullshit: talk nonsense to someone in an attempt to deceive them, or use stupid or untrue talk.

Trying to condense this down is near to impossible. Phone calls were made, emails sent from my lawyer to me, and even a long letter from me back to my lawyer. This is all going down in the last five working days before my lawyer closed up for his Christmas break, and I have to admit I did throw a bit of a tantrum when I read what the insurance company came back with when I said that I wanted my "pocket money" paid before my lawyer closed his doors. Yeah, definitely a tantrum, and as I was doing this I knew it wasn't going to happen and that I really had no right to expect this of my lawyer regardless of what might happen next. My lawyer and his team are terrific but I know they can't do the impossible even though I have seen my lawyer magically pull the Human Resources Manager out of thin air! Always knew those slippery little suckers were hiding out in Sydney somewhere.

I will try to convey what happened next as if all was done in one "to" phone call/email/letter and one "fro" phone call/email/letter. My lawyer has spoken to the insurance company which I will refer to as "that mob" in the following, and below is what my lawyer was advised and my thoughts on it:

That Mob: Say they received an email on the 12th of December 2013 at 4:06pm stating that the appointment had been cancelled. My appointment had been set for 5:15pm, OBSTACLE 36.

That mob continued to say that the recipient of that email had left their office for the day, OBSTACLE 37.

251

And that they did not receive a phone call from the doctor's surgery advising of the cancellation, OBSTACLE 38.

That mob then stated that the doctor's Surgery require ten days notice whether a person will be attending an appointment or not, OBSTACLE 39.

That mob advised us that they had not been told that there was a ten-day notice required. LIE, oops I mean, OBSTACLE 40.

My Lawyer: Told that mob that we were informed that there was a five-day notice period for confirmation which was abided by. My Lawyer told them again that this was completely unacceptable to which that mob agreed, and apparently that mob is very apologetic for the distress that was caused to me and also expressed their "sincere" apologies for the inconvenience caused.

My lawyer then went on to say that they acknowledge and understand my frustrations with processing my claim to date, which was appreciated.

Me: Firstly I advised my lawyer that I didn't care for that mob's apologies, excuses or whatevers. I then asked if we could get a copy of that email that that mob were saying they received, as what that was stating to my lawyer was contradicting what the two receptionists had told me. I also told him that I believe that mob didn't receive a phone call in regard to the cancellation as there was no appointment booked to cancel.

As for that mob saying they had no knowledge of the ten-day notice, that was ludicrous in itself. So this would mean that mob didn't have any real communication with this dermatologist, as the dermatologist has cancelled it due to me not abiding by his ten day period, one hour and nine minutes before I was to attend? So how was he to know I had confirmed attendance? Didn't that mob advise him I had confirmed my attendance on the 5th of December? Well I reckon he didn't need to know as no appointment had been booked for me!

And another thing, if this mob is claiming that the dermatologist cancelled it one hour and nine minutes before I was due to arrive, why hadn't this dermatologist abided by his own rules and cancelled it earlier? By his ten days I should have confirmed on the 28th Nov 2013, by that mob's instructions I was to confirm on the 5th December 2013.

Looking at this logically, if that is at all possible, he had a good five days prior to cancel it as we didn't abide by his ten-day rule, but he didn't until one hour and nine minutes before I was to turn up? Getting confused yet? Yeah what a crock of crap! If you are going to lie you have to be good at it and have a good memory because lies and deceit don't stick like the truth does. Once again I say to that mob, the truth is definitely not negotiable, regardless of who you try to blame or how underhanded you try to be.

Oh, and as it turned out the supposed email received at 4:06pm, stating that the cancellation actually was two hours and nine minutes before I was due to arrive, as that mob is on daylight saving time and is one hour ahead of us here in Queensland. Does it matter? I don't know.

I then said to my lawyer, "This is what I reckon; that mob are liable for this mess and are fully aware of it. An appointment was never made for me by that mob on the 12th December 2013. There is no supposed email, and if the email does materialize, well I will be going through it with a fine toothed comb." I ended this part of this mess telling my lawyer that I am not attending any more appointments set by the insurance company, I am over being treated like a moron and I am not proving to anyone again how debilitating this journey has been and continues to be for me. Soon enough another email was received from my lawyer stating the insurance company had set another date for me to see the dermatologist on the 17th of January 2014, this now being another five weeks away, OBSTACLE 41.

Just to remind you, it is only a few sleeps away until my lawyer is on his Christmas break. "No I will not be attending the new appointment," was my reply.

Funnily enough, the insurance company can get back to us quicker than the speed of light with an appointment when it suits them! So to me, this confirms that they didn't try to bring the first "dropped in the big black hole of bullshit," appointment forward. Oi! Hang on a minute! What am I saying? That appointment didn't even exist! Aren't I a silly middle-aged menopausal woman for getting confused over all that! It also proves they didn't try to change it as if they had, they would have learnt of this error. Hmm, it proves that there was no appointment booked for me on the 12th of December 2013, and it also proves the lack of communication that the insurance company had with the dermatologist's surgery. Bingo!

Yeah, that's right insurance company I've got my eye on you lot. I still don't get why they booked me in on the 9th of December without advising me or my solicitor, or why they then went ahead and just cancelled it. They're not even clever with their fibs. Now, three sleeps away from my lawyer going on holiday, I get a call from one of my lawyers' teams asking me to confirm attendance. I once again confirmed that no, I was not attending, that the insurance company is fully aware of what went down and this would now mean my claim will sit dormant for a good three months.

I then received an email from my lawyer saying that they understood my "had enough" attitude and can only recommend I do attend the re-scheduled appointment, and as they were closing for holidays in three sleeps, they wanted it confirmed with the insurance company beforehand to ensure all times frames are met. In the back of my mind I knew I would go, I didn't want to "cut my nose off to spite my face." Anyway that mob might be just waiting for this response so they can collect that $1000 bucks off me, as yes, that condition still stands.

Two sleeps before my lawyer's holidays I shot an email off confirming my attendance. The main reason I changed my mind about going though, was that I owed it to my loved ones. Also I don't ever recall having a conversation with my lawyer that he was happy to be paid in buttons for his fee. On top of that, I haven't got the energy to start gathering 1000 buttons for that mob as payment if I don't attend. One sleep before my lawyer's doors closed for holiday, I received an email from him saying that the appointment had been confirmed with that mob.

So, everyone now confused and exhausted reading all of that? Basically my claim is now sitting dormant for three months. Yep, the new allergist's report went in on October 2013 and now I have to wait until January 2014 to attend this re-scheduled appointment. Is this legally allowed? I pay this insurance cover for when it is needed and it is needed now, but the insurance company seemed to be allowed to say and do whatever they want. I just don't get it. In a very small, very minute way, I am glad that my lawyer has had another taste of what I have had to deal with throughout this journey.

I have a feeling that he and his team are going to be ready to pounce legally in 2014. I also know I have one main question to ask this dermatologist when I see him and that is, "Why did you cancel my appointment two hours and nine minutes before I was due to attend?" My gut feeling is telling me he isn't going to know anything about it.

All this is now finally being hung up six sleeps before Christmas Day 2013. What can I say? We have Christmas coming up, then my birthday, then New Years Eve. I am putting it all to bed and once again am going to enjoy this time with my loved ones as well as my health will allow. Wow, I remember saying that earlier, this time though I will also be singing "All I want for Christmas is my one front tooth." Yeah, it's a cute look when you are first losing your baby teeth, not so cute when you are fifty-two. Oh well I have mastered the art of mumble and could give Marcel Marceau, may he rest in peace, a run for his money in regard to mime.

Throughout all the dealings with the insurance company and my lawyer in regard to that mob, I kept thinking about what my BHRT doctor said about my headaches, that yes, coming down off the steroids would play a part in them, but also having too much BHRT progesterone could be a reason too. You know overdosing myself with the BHRT proves that it is working! I remember when I had been on it just under three weeks and my energy level was a bit better. Was this when I had the right amount of BHRT in me?

So even though I have overdosed, I know it is working, I felt it! We have fine-tuned it again and I am happy to say the headaches have eased. Wow, I must admit the headaches were starting to feel like the HRT headaches, but unlike HRT, with BHRT not one drop of blood have I had to lose. Even with this overdosing, I have done no damage as it is all natural and plant based, and unlike HRT I can keep tweaking the amount of natural progesterone level my body needs until it is totally fine-tuned to my individual needs. I know I am not even close to being the healthy and strong one I used to be but, I yam what I yam and this excites me. Merry Christmas everyone, here's to 2014 being a much healthier, happier and less stressful year. Surely the worst of it is all behind me and I get to just concentrate on my health. We will see. For now enjoy! Oh and metal note to self: I forgot to ask my lawyer if this now means the insurance company owes *me* a thousand bucks for just purely screwing me around? Hmm I wonder. Ok. Back at you all in 2014.

Chapter 41

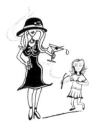

HAPPY NEW YEAR IT IS NOW 2014

So a new year has arrived and to be honest the whole thought of it exhausts me. I know that sounds very negative and dramatic, but I just feel like my whole life force is seeping away. Maybe I am still just tired from that crock of crap that went down with the insurance company. Anyway, Christmas was lovely, but of course an incident happened. Our beautiful dog who is quite old hasn't been well and has been on medication for a cough. It was getting worse so she needed a trip to the vet, but the old girl had no intention of going. I ended up having a chat to her vet over the phone and we decided to try another form of medication which has helped. The vet also had *that* chat to me, so we are keeping an eye on the old girl. No, not me, I am middle-aged, and if that time is coming… well, we will wait and see.

It's a really hard place to be when you know one day you might have to make that decision in regard to a pet. We love her and don't want her to go, but we don't want to prolong the suffering either. Each Christmas Day our dog has a stocking with doggy goodies in it. The daughter went down to give our dog a doggy treat and the next minute I heard

"Muuum!" I went down to see the dog lying down and my daughter kneeling in front of her sobbing, "Get up Ginger!" I tell you it was gut wrenching. The daughter was upset and the dog wouldn't get up.

The daughter went to give her a treat but I said make her walk to it. And so she did. What had upset my daughter is that the dog was trying to get the daughter to hold her paw, yes she likes her paw held, which the daughter knows, but the daughter thought the dog was struggling to get up. You know I was watching all this - and what I am about to say I know is horrible - but while I'm watching this I was thinking, "Yeah that would be right. Go on! Pass over on Christmas Day dog. Why not, it's been a shit of a year again health wise, why not add to it with you passing over on bloody Christmas Day!" Horrible I know but geez all mighty!

I'm glad to say though that the dog has improved heaps. She still demands her breakfast, lunch and dinner, and still gallops towards us like a pup on occasion. Sad to say we still have to keep an eye on her as we know her time is coming. We have her vet organized to come here as this is our dog's home, but I am really praying that we don't have to make that decision. I pray that she just passes away in her sleep knowing how much love she gave us and how much we loved her back. I can guarantee though that my adrenal glands, which I will nickname A1 and A2, were looking at each other after that scare thinking, "Well with all the stresses around this menopausal woman, we have no bloody hope! It's been great working with you A1." "Yeah back at yar A2. Oi and kidneys, thanks for letting us sloth on you both for all these years!"

My birthday was lovely, nothing big as I haven't got the health or energy, but I was very spoilt and now here we are in the New Year.

I have that dermatologist appointment looming and it got me thinking. What is the difference between an allergist and a dermatologist? This is what I found: A dermatologist is a qualified medical specialist who specialises in the diagnosis and treatment of skin diseases and cancers, whereas an allergist is a medical doctor who specialises in the diagnosis and treatment of various allergic diseases such as asthma and conditions of the immune system. The latter speaks to me.

So. Why am I being sent to see this dermatologist? I think this is just another prime example of how no one knows where to put the menopausal woman or, maybe the Insurance Company is just trying to delay the inevitable, and that is paying out my bloody claim!

So to sum up I have been with my doctor since the start of my acquaintance with Ms Menopause in 2010. I have now seen two allergists who have both seen fit to treat me differently, medically. I am in the care of my BHRT doctor and they now want me to see a dermatologist?

Let us not forget the endocrinologist who was lovely but really had nothing for me heath wise, and oh yes, the psychologist who was willing to stick me on anti-depressants even though he wasn't sure why I was dealing with depression. This just proves to me that no one knows where to put the menopausal woman and no one knows how to treat the menopausal woman medically in a safe way, except you my BHRT doc!

Plus the insurance company is a big liar! Yeah, that definitely feels like it has gone from David and Goliath to just me, my lawyer and his team against the whole bloody establishment. Maybe this is also why I am starting this New Year exhausted.

I am also supposed to have gone down to 7mg of steroids but I can feel my body is struggling on 8mg. I am seeing more flare ups in my skin so I am not game enough to go down to 7mg until I get on those adrenal herbs. The body produces, well actually, the adrenal glands produce cortisone naturally, and this is the time we are waiting to see if my adrenal glands kick back in and start producing their own again. Due to the insurance company doing what they did, it has delayed the payment date of my claim. My loved ones are wonderful. It was decided that I am at a critical stage with my health. Ok, I really need to rephrase that sentence. I am at a critical stage in regard to my adrenal glands, so funds are being taken from wherever I can find them so I that can see my BHRT doctor in the last week of January and get started on the adrenal herbs.

I just noticed I haven't even mentioned Ms Menopause at all in this New Year yet, but I sit here in 2014 at fifty-three, a middle-aged woman with, they say, a mental disorder, an immune system which is attacking itself and exhausted adrenal glands. Wow who would have thought the loss of these two hormones could do so much damage to a woman.

I have also been thinking about those women who have "sailed" through menopause. The more I hear and read, the more it seems that while these women may sail through menopause or not have too much of a hard time, they end up dealing with "old-age" illnesses just as much as those who don't sail through it. For example, of three women I know who said that menopause wasn't too bad for them, one now deals with osteoporosis, another with bruising if she merely gently knocks her skin, and now she has had problems with her shoulder for the last few months and has had to have a steroid shot to ease it, while the other is dealing with a cancer in her nose.

I also recently spoke to a woman who is five years into her menopause. This woman said that the hot flushes and night sweats aren't too bad for her but she is now starting to get aching and soreness throughout her body. She also said that she has seen a few of her friends suffer quite a bit with their menopause. Look I know that as we get older our bodies start to deteriorate, that's natural. And I know that other health issues may arise that have nothing to do with Ms Menopause, but I've found through my limited research that not much happens to women during menopause and beyond without her input.

Oh, and to the medical world, I'm not stupid, but the age range of these women I have just spoken about is from fifty to seventy with the mid-fifties being the average age. These women should not be feeling the effects of old age in their mid fifties, they are in their middle age. The seventy-year old woman I spoke to is a very strong Irish woman who has worked all her life. This woman originally told me that menopause wasn't that bad for her, but I need to get back to her as I remember her telling me she tried HRT but she too bled all the way through it. But if menopause wasn't too bad for her why the need for HRT? I am really starting to believe that women who feel as if they have to suffer in silence are the ones that may feel that they also have to say that menopause wasn't that bad for them. Or maybe that's just how they want to do their menopause which is their right.

Back to the strong Irish woman with the bruising and the arthritis which is being treated with steroid shots for the pain. This woman has been the matriarch of her family, raising her children and then doing it all again with her grandchildren. I talk to her and see that she is not well, but her bruising is not from being on long term steroids as the steroid shot she had to have was done after her bruising had started. Her bruising would be from the loss of collagen in her body resulting from menopause, as a lack of collagen also causes thinning of the blood vessels in our bodies.

I really don't believe this woman would be dealing with these ills at seventy if she'd been educated about menopause twenty odd years ago when she started her "not too bad" menopause. I know there will be some who may think that seventy is old and that this seventy year old is just deteriorating naturally due to old age, but I disagree. There is no need for this strong seventy year old to be feeling the effects of perhaps her eighties while still in her seventies. I used to be sincerely happy for those women who say they sailed through menopause or that it wasn't too bad for them. I now worry for them as due to my long battle with Ms Menopause I have come to realize that no one actually sails through menopause. If Ms Menopause doesn't get you at the beginning or in the middle of your journey, she definitely gets you at the end of it.

Women around the world will feel and deal with the symptoms of Ms Menopause whether it is in the early years of her arrival or later down the track. Regardless of whether we suffer through it or sail through it, we all suffer the loss of those hormones. It has been said that a woman spends one third of her life dealing with menopause, but I believe it is more than one third so, as an example only, if we look at eighty-five being our life span, this means from the average age of fifty women start their menopause. Fabulous, thirty-five odd years of Ms Menopause and beyond! Feckin dandy! Then as the years go by, menopause gets called and is being allowed to become, other illnesses and diseases.

By this time though, Ms Menopause has well and truly packed her bags and moved on leaving women being told that menopause has nothing to do with their health problems, that it is just due to old age, and then being put on all sorts of medications which could have been avoided if - here comes my catch cry - we had the truth and education at the very beginning.

Do I want and expect to live forever? Hell no! I like the cycle of life. Do I want and expect to be young forever? Nah. Been there, done that. What I do want and expect is to be able to live to the end of my natural life feeling healthy, happy and me. Women who have been strong, healthy, able women all their lives should not be rapidly deteriorating once Ms Menopause knocks on their doors but it is being allowed. I came across the "frozen shoulder" in my research. Apparently many Japanese women suffer with this when they reach menopause. It is also known in Japan as the "fifties shoulder". It is said to be very painful, the muscles feel like concrete and it is impossible to lift the arm. Frozen shoulder is also known at times as menopause tendonitis or arthritis.

I read an article about a woman who suffered for ages due to two doctors dismissing the idea of this being hormonal. Once she was treated with hormone replacement therapy her frozen shoulder started to ease and the woman claimed, "I would never, ever have thought that simple "hormones" could cause so much pain and ruin my life. Menopause changed me from being a fairly fit fifty year old into a crippled ninety year old." I am hearing you sister!

So heading back to my seventy year old Irish friend, I believe she is now suffering with a frozen shoulder caused by menopause, but of course the doctors straight away inject her with steroids and put it all down to old age. I also know now that these, estrogen and progesterone, are not "simple" hormones. They are the two big kahoona hormones that keep a woman healthy in life right through from puberty to menopause.

Imagine the amounts of medications needed by more mature menopausal women, oh that's right, by then it is all put down to aging.

Take me for example. If I had taken everything that I was advised to take during my menopausal time I would today be on sleeping tablets, anti-depressants, inflammation suppressant medication used to stop rejection of organs in transplant patients and perhaps still on HRT, ooh shiver! Now add that to the steroids I have lived on since 2011, the antibiotics I have had to live on at times and sometimes for months, the steroid creams and all those desensitization injections. I have mentioned all the other bits and pieces of drugs I have had. Wow what a flaming even bigger mess I would be in today.

I know I was born with a few allergies, but they only worsened a little bit after my pregnancy and as we all know I am just one big allergy ball on legs now, with an immune system which is attacking itself all thanks to menopause, so it is all hormonal.

I wonder now if all that crap about keeping us in the dark about menopause is purely for the pharmaceutical companies to keep making their profits. HRT is a billion dollar business and I am sure millions of menopausal women contribute to the profits of these companies in other ways by needing all sorts of other medications for all sorts of menopause-related illnesses in their later life, so yeah, again I say, "You Ms Menopause are a gigantic money making machine."

It also never made sense to me that by not educating us about menopause, they have put a bigger strain on our heath care system, but I think I get it now.

The lack of education and transparency creates an escalation into other illnesses and diseases, which in turn require huge amounts of extra medications, which end up costing us huge amounts of money with the end result being huge amounts of profit for the pharmaceutical companies.

I will also say doing it naturally isn't cheap either, but why do I still have to go to a doctor to get a script for the natural medications I want to put in my body? They say natural medicines are not scientifically proven but they still treat them like other medications in that we have to get a prescription. Well this proves to me that they know that natural methods work. It is just another way that the pharmaceutical companies protect their profits and control those of us who want to get better our way.

Why are these natural remedies so expensive and put out of the reach of many people who choose to do their healing naturally, and that's not only the menopausal woman. The answer always comes back to the dollars that these big companies make. Who gave them, whoever them is, the right to take our right away to use natural methods? Some say they haven't taken our right away as we are able to obtain the natural medications. Yeah right, have you seen the cost of them? There needs to be more natural medications listed on our PBS so people from all walks of life get the right to survival and good health even if they haven't got big money in the bank.

Ok, time to step down from my invisible soapbox and head off to see the dermatologist at the insurance company's request. I felt I was more mentally and emotionally prepared this second time round and really didn't feel all that stressed. Well what's the point of stressing out over it now that the company has taken fair play off the table? I was more prepared with notes and photos too. Yeah, photos. I decided this time I would gather any photos taken of me during this journey. It was interesting to look back over them. All I could say to a loved one as we were gathering what photos we did have was, "Geez I've suffered, haven't I?" I know I have and am still fighting for my health and wellbeing, but it makes it even more real when you have photos of it.

I wish now I had documented my whole journey with photos, but I didn't know what was coming. More photos are being taken now since I realized the insurance company is messing me around. My advice to you all is, document your journey with photos and write it all down just in case you need it one day. Oh wait a minute, all you girls will be ok as you all know now to get on top of Ms Menopause earlier as you now have the truth and education and know all your options. Yahoo! I was thinking how I should have documented my journey, but then I realized I already have, through these writings! I never ever thought about this as being a form of evidence if needed, it is only now since that insurance mob did what they did that I realise how important this book may be in other ways as well. We shall wait and see but for now I continue to write in the hope it benefits my daughter and all women.

Another thing I must say in regard to this dermatologist is, ok I got it wrong! From what I've discovered you don't have a previous relationship with the insurance company and this is not a little money-spinner for you, so I am sorry for even thinking it. This dermatologist is quite a bigwig in his field and is even a director of a department for dermatology at a large hospital and also lectures on dermatology to other specialists. I must say I liked him, he was very down to earth, but then again I have seen other bigwigs with a nice manner throughout this journey who still do not know, or who choose not to know, the real Ms Menopause and what she is capable of.

So we started. We went through it all, photos were looked at, and the dermatologist took photos of me and me skin. I had to smile, no not for the camera, but the way he was hiding from me what he was reading by cupping his hand around the questions he was asking. I then asked him if those were the questions from the insurance company. He said yes but he couldn't really understand some of them. Yeah, I thought to myself, I bet those questions are phrased in a way that no answer I give will benefit me! I also noticed the file he had on me was huge. Where did that all come from? Please God, please let it be my file and not another me's file. Thank you.

The end result was that in his professional opinion I have been mismanaged all the way throughout my journey, yay, and that I should have been seeing a dermatologist from the start, hmmm, ok. And he was going to recommend I now see a dermatologist, boo! Even though he did agree with me that this might have all started with Ms Menopause, he feels all my problems are due to the steroids I have been on and he feels I could do with ultraviolet light therapy. I am just staring at him now hearing nothing but CRICKETS!

Don't get me wrong, I agree and fully understand the effects that the long term steroids have had on me but I had to remind him that my health started to deteriorate with Ms Menopause a year before I was put on steroids. He also listed off about five symptoms of side effects from the steroids and when he finished all I could say was they are all symptoms of menopause as well. No joking, all the symptoms he rattled off about steroids were exact symptoms of menopause.

I wondered later if he was trying to say that menopause doesn't even exist and that the steroids have caused all the problems, even though earlier he seemed to agree that this may have started with menopause. Nah, maybe not because I know I was affected by Ms Menopause a good year before those little suckers, steroids that is, even came into my life! So no, surely not! Oh my god, I need to stop thinking about it as it is becoming a more "probable" thought that maybe the dermatologist was "subtly" trying to convey this to me. I guess it will be wait and see when we get his report.

Not picking up on his "maybe" subtle opinion, I went on to let him know how I want to be treated and that is with BHRT, which he didn't know about, and with adrenal herbs. When we finished he advised me that his report would be into the insurance company in two weeks. When I got home I realized I had notes of everyday things I deal with that I had forgotten to give him. It is so different living "it" daily to having to sit down and try to relate all of "it" in one appointment, so the next working day I popped the notes in to a receptionist to put in my file for him to read. I also explained in these notes that I want to be monitored by my BHRT doctor. I said that I agree with him that I have been mismanaged all the way through this, but there doesn't seem to be anyone who does know how to manage the menopausal woman, or maybe they do and they are just choosing not to manage us in a way that they should be. I hope he doesn't dare to put in his report that this has nothing to do with Ms Menopause, because if he does, well I won't like him much! Actually it won't matter much if he does as I have all the proof I need that this is Ms Menopause's doing and that proof is me!

Before I had left this appointment I also asked him what one of the blood results meant. He told me he didn't know what it meant "for me". Ok, I understand he needs time to look it all over but that was a bit curious to me. Does that mean two people can have the same blood test done which come back with the same results but the results may have a different meaning depending on the person? Huh? I don't know, I am but a layperson so hopefully that is explained in his report which I will be getting a copy of. At least, I thought, he is being thorough and not just giving me any old answer, I think.

Regardless of that, I liked him. He was very thorough and professional. I did listen to what he was saying and I could tell that he was really wanting to get to the bottom of my health issues but once again I walked away from one of these professionals who are at the top of the food chain within their chosen field, thinking, yeahnah! With great and deserved respect to this dermatologist, it just goes to show that there are no professionals who are experts in menopause. The only professional I am putting my faith in is my BHRT doctor and I believe he is the one who is closest to an expert on menopause that I have met throughout this whole journey.

Oh that's right let's get to the exciting bit. Yes I asked the dermatologist that question. You know, the "Why did you cancel my appointment in December, two hours and nine minutes before I was due to attend?" I didn't phrase it exactly like that but when I told him I had rocked up for that appointment with him in December, he looked down at the ground confused, shaking his head while trying to figure it out. He then walked back to his desk, checked something and confirmed that no appointment had been made for me to see him on the 12th of December 2013.

I did say to him that, no, I didn't think he had cancelled it, and I let him know that my lawyer received an email from the insurance company saying that he had cancelled it. This dermatologist had the right to know that the insurance company was pointing the finger at him for their mix up. So not only has the insurance company lied to my lawyer and me, they also had the hide to try and put the blame on this dermatologist. All I'm thinking now is, "Find the loophole my wonderful lawyer."

I also said to him as I was walking out that if I do see a dermatologist I would like to see him, but unfortunately because he is doing the report for the insurance company, he can't treat me. Oh well, it's not a biggie because I am not seeing a dermatologist. That's right! Done and dusted now! I know how I want to be treated and it's time to dig the heels in again. I don't believe the insurance company has the right to tell me how I try to get my health back, so they can feck off!

I sent emails to my lawyer letting him know I'd been to the appointment and another asking him to ensure that the insurance company has the details of my BHRT doctor, as that is who I want to be treated and monitored by. Yes I will still see my second allergist, but have put that back to March and will keep my own doctor in the loop, but I will not let that insurance company dictate who I must see and how I must treat my symptoms.

If anything I was doing was detrimental to my health like being on HRT, sleeping tablets, anti-depressants, super dooper immune suppressant drugs, hmmm have I forgotten anything, or if I just wasn't trying, then maybe I could understand them having a say but again, the way I want to be treated and who I want to monitor me is, as far as I am concerned, the best way for me. Oh and also it's my feckin right!

So again I say, and with much passion, to the insurance company, feck off! I have nada respect for you now after you telling those huge fibs. You sit there trying to hold on to dollars that I am entitled to without a care as to how my loved ones and I are affected. It's honestly beyond me how these big establishments are allowed to do this. Oh and now because the dermatologist has been given two weeks to send his report in, my claim will now sit dormant for one week short of four months, and who knows how much time you will take to action the report! Geez my stress levels go up just writing about it!

When I was pondering the conversation between the dermatologist and me, I thought about his comment that I should have been seeing a dermatologist from the start. In the material from the first allergist, he had stated that he strongly suggested that I see a dermatologist. When I read that I thought, "That's news to me!" I don't recall my own doctor talking to me about seeing a dermatologist, but if he has and I have just forgotten, well I am sure it is in his records. When I was admitted to hospital in 2012 swollen and inflamed with my head, as my daughter said, "three times its size," and "Clancy" the nurse "sticking it to me" trying to get my blood, one of the medical team there suggested a dermatologist and even though I tried to tell her this was all purely due to menopause, my words were dismissed and she booked me into the public hospital system with an appointment.

This brings up a thought. I wrote earlier about that hospital stay and also how I questioned the doctor as to why I had to have two lots of blood taken. Her reply was that the first lot of blood results looked "scary" but this "error" can happen because of the way the blood is taken at times. The second lot of bloods didn't come back scary, or I assume not. Now I wonder if the first bloods were actually a true indication of what I was dealing with. By the time they took the second lot of bloods I was pumped up with a higher dose of steroids. I was on that drug that made me feel fabulous, and I was also on something else. So now I really wonder if that first blood result was right and not just scary due to human error in the taking of the blood. I don't know.

Later down the track, I cancelled the appointment with the public hospital dermatologist as I was days away from seeing my allergist. Why would I need to see a dermatologist if my problem is menopause and the inflammation and swelling is due to the loss of those two hormones? Well I reckon that dermatologist would not even have had an answer for that back then. Looking back on it, why the hell was I seeing an allergist who dismissed my menopause? There is no need for me, a menopausal woman, to be tied into the public hospital system, geez almighty! Actually none of this matters now, except for that first blood test result which I am more curious about now, but this far up the track I'm not seeing a dermatologist, so that's that!

With a new year started I have been thinking lately that I never had a problem getting older but I have to admit I am starting to resent the years Ms Menopause has stolen from me heath wise. I started this journey mid 2010 when I was forty-nine and had my last period in the month of my fiftieth birthday. I had to walk from my job mid 2012 when I was fifty-one and I have just turned fifty-three so yeah, time is moving on and not having my health so far all the way through my fifties, I have felt a lot older than I should be feeling. It also makes me feel sad. I am so far away from that time when I believed that my fifties were going to be my best years. Oh well it's time now to see my BHRT doctor.

You know I don't think I have ever told you how clever he is. He has a special interest in women's health, this on top of his regular general practice work. He also specialises in BHRT and in many chronic illnesses such as fibromyalgia, diabetes, osteoporosis, arthritis, fatigue and a range of gastro-intestinal diseases. He works within the framework of integrative medicine using both conventional medication and a broad range of complimentary and natural therapies.

In the past he has lectured at a college of acupuncture and natural therapies and was the Chairman of that college. He currently teaches and educates in a university and has given my daughter her health back by using natural methods. She is now back on her feet and back into her life. She is happy and able and is also earning pretty damn good dollars again as well. If we had stayed with the conventional medicine, I hate to think of the damage the long-term use of those super dooper antibiotics could have had on my baby!

As soon as I was slumped in my BHRT doctor's chair I announced that I was done with all the rest and that I wanted to work with and be monitored by him. We then got into it all. He had previously contacted pathology and was advised that as I was on steroids there was no point doing a test for Addison's disease as it would give a false reading, so that is on the back burner. I am to start my adrenal tablets to help with getting off the steroids, as for natural oestrogen we are just waiting to see if this will be needed a little further down the track. I did say to him that even though I am having a few flare-ups with my skin I really felt that the BHRT is "holding" me. He agreed that yes it would be, as progesterone is an anti-inflammatory hormone. Wow, that was news to me and was very exciting to hear.

This was really interesting. We know through tests that I had no progesterone in my body which is the norm when dealing with Ms Menopause, and I know now that progesterone is an anti-

271

inflammatory hormone. Since the onset of menopause I have been having inflammation and swelling, so there you go, my own scientific proof that all my health issues are due to Ms Menopause. I know they are, I just wanted to put it in print.

He then said that he would like to do a biopsy of my skin where the discolouration is. Yeah, the skin on my arms from my wrist to my elbow is now darker.

Before I continue with my BHRT doc's conversation, there have been a few professional opinions as to why my skin is discoloured. We know it all started with bruising and bleeding from being on long term steroids, but I also know now it can be due to the loss of collagen we experience during menopause. Ok, firstly my doctor told me it was iron left under my skin from the bumping and bleeding. I can't remember whether the first allergist had an opinion on it but I would say that he didn't because I would have remembered that, as no doubt it would have been something ludicrous. The second allergist said it was purely due to the long-term use of steroids. The dermatologist I had to see said it was caused by sun damage and long-term steroid use. I did question him on the sun damage but he's the professional, I'm just the patient, and he was adamant that it was also sun damage. When I told my BHRT doctor that the dermatologist thought it was sun damaged he disagreed.

So there we go, I know that steroids are quite consistently blamed, but once again there are a few different opinions as to why my skin is now discoloured. I don't expect the medical mob to have an instant answer for me every time I see them but I would expect them to go away and find out. I also know they have to cover their own backsides legally, but what I would expect is that they are all on the same page as to how to treat me, and I also would expect one united answer as to the cause of my skin discolouration. Is this just another example of the medical world not knowing how to properly treat a menopausal woman? I say definitely they have no idea how to look after "moi"! Anyhoo time to head back to that conversation with my BHRT doc.

Doc: We will do a biopsy and take some skin to get it tested. It will only require one stitch once it is done.
Me: ONE STITCH?

Feckin hell! I was terrified when he mentioned the word "stitch." The only time I have ever had stitches was after giving birth to my daughter twenty-two years ago, but let's not forget I was whisked away to surgery pretty quickly and pretty well "non compos mentis," and I had no idea what was going on until my loved ones were relieved to see me still breathing and the doctors let me know what had happened, plus I was on pretty good "knock me out drugs" for those stitches. Geez almighty! Oh and geez sorry doc. Can't have any stitches until I go down in steroids as I haven't got good healing skin yet, oh what a shame! We agreed to do it, maybe, when I am on a lower amount of steroids and when I feel a little stronger. I'm personally not in any hurry for that to go down!

Just a little memory of that time: I found out later that my family was waiting for me while I was in surgery. When they heard I was being wheeled back to my room they all gathered around the lifts to be there for me. Apparently, my sister told me later, when the lift doors opened I was chatting away to the two male doctors who had brought me down and they were in stitches laughing! Oh dear! I never had a chance to ask them what I was saying, but looking back on it, maybe it was a good thing I didn't know. I know I reckon I have a pretty good sense of humour, but unfortunately this time I think I have to give the drugs I was on some of the credit.

Anyhoo, back to now. The BHRT doctor still wants me to see my allergist and as much as I said I am "done", I let my BHRT doctor know that I am booked in to see my new allergist again in March, and then we went on and had a good chat. You know, besides the "stitch" thing, and how he scared me once by the urgency in his voice after which I walked straight out and saw that four car smash, I always walk away from my appointments with him feeling better and with hope by my side. I always feel a little lighter with everything I am dealing with as I know he is the closest thing to an expert on menopause that I am going to meet. I have been through a lot to get to him and to this point.

So where am I now? Well it is January 2014. I have now been on my adrenal tablets for seven days. I had to build up to four a day and have. I've gone down to 7mg of steroids in the last three days and am stable. I am still on my BHRT which we are still fine-tuning to my individual needs, but I am not suffering with severe headaches so we are getting there. I know I still have a long way to go as it's going to take until at least August 2014 to be off steroids all together and that will depend on whether I have any sick days and have to increase the steroids, but I'm thinking I will be ok now.

I know I need to start walking again to strengthen my mind, body and soul and also to tone up this extra 10-15kg of weight I now carry around. Don't get me wrong I am a great believer that women look sexier with curves, skinny is not a shape for me, but I don't feel healthy with this extra weight on. But I also understand the bloating of menopause itself and the fatty liver I now have due to the steroids isn't helping. Ooh that's right I still need to get my front tooth back, but have to wait to see how my body reacts to being on 7mg and lower of steroids. I am still tired and some days just plain exhausted. As for my financial status, well to be honest if it wasn't for the loved ones I don't know where I would be today. All the love and support my little tribe has given me unconditionally all the way through this mess is very much appreciated. I am very grateful and feel very blessed. They have had to go without things many times throughout this journey, but they just want me to get better. That is very humbling and wonderful. I do know that as much as I want to "be" for me, my fight for survival has been even stronger because of the love I have for these special people. Oooh! Where are the tissues?

I also need to say that I feel like my body has breathed a sigh of relief, a feeling of "finally we are getting there". All my senses feel like they are squealing with excitement at the thought that we are all going to be ok. I know it's still early days, and we may still be dealing with Addison's disease, but yeah, my mind, body and soul is talking to me and I like the feel of what they are saying. As for my adrenal glands, A1 and A2, I think they are the most excited. I used to say, "some days are diamond, some days are stone," when asked in the early stages how I was. I really now need to remember that "some days are stone, some days are pebbles" where it all could fall to pieces again, but I'm going to keep the faith and have faith in my BHRT doctor.

Ok, now this is what I wrote next, but after seeing my BHRT doc again at the end of February I walked away from him thinking to myself, "Jen you are a moron!" Why? Well I will tell you once you read the following. This is originally what I wrote:

This is my hope as the countdown is on: 7,6,5,4,3,2,1, zero steroids as my adrenal glands, A1 and A2 are healthy and happy again producing our body's own natural steroid. My immune system goes back to normal, as the BHRT progesterone is an anti-inflammatory hormone among other things. I go back to having one or two minor allergies which have been a part of me from birth, oh ok being allergic to housework isn't a "born with" allergy. I am only on BHRT long term and my body's network is healthy, happy and chatting to each other again by being that remarkable finely tuned network that it is.

Now all of the above still stands in my head but... My wonderful brother celebrated his fiftieth the weekend before I was due to see my BHRT doc. Of course there were yummy foods to celebrate this wonderful day. I was careful with what I ate but I really needed to have little nibbles and some birthday cake! In the following few days my skin flared up a bit once again and how it makes me feel inside is really hard to explain. At my appointment with my BHRT doc we discussed this flare up and I told him that it could be a bit self-inflicted. He said that self-inflicted would be the better option.

We talked about how I am still reacting to stuff quite fast, even though I am still doing better on a day-to-day basis. We agreed to increase my adrenal tablets from four to six a day to see if this improves my energy level. I was to go down to 6mg of steroids the next day but my BHRT doc wants me to stay on 7mg for an extra week due to this flare up, and we have upped the BHRT.

Now this is when the "I am a moron" bit comes in. While talking to my BHRT doctor about adrenal gland exhaustion he told me that it will take a good twelve to eighteen months more before A1 and A2 will be working by themselves again. You know as he said this and while he was organizing another script for my adrenal tablets, I sat there thinking, "I have already written about this time frame, so why did I think that A1 and A2 would just bounce back after getting to zero synthetic steroids? Jen you are a moron! You need to re-read everything you have written!"

Hopefully A1 and A2 are just exhausted because if they aren't and my body shows signs of A1 and A2 karking it once I am off the synthetic steroids, then that would mean I have Addison's disease which will require me to be on medication for the rest of my life.

Once home and after the loved ones had been told what was happening I went and sat by myself and just pondered it all. I actually felt a bit overwhelmed with the twelve to eighteen months bit. I know I had just said that I always walk away with hope by my side after seeing my BHRT doctor, and I still do, but I have to admit I kept thinking to myself, "I don't know if I can do another twelve to eighteen months of this. I don't know if I have the courage, energy or strength to do another twelve to eighteen months of THIS!

I felt that my loved ones were disheartened by this timeframe too, they are also tired. I know I have said that I am the one physically going through menopause but my loved ones have been there for me every step of the way through this journey. They must be tired and losing hope that I will get to the end of this.

But I have also noticed in the days after seeing my BHRT doctor that I am a bit sniffly, am sneezing a wee bit more, and have just had a wee bit of congestion on my chest which I have never had to deal with throughout this journey, so perhaps this set-back wasn't all totally self-inflicted, maybe I have the rumblings of a bit of a cold coming on. I know this doesn't change the twelve to eighteen month timeframe and that still feels too big right now, but a cold added to my "nibbles" could have made everything appear worse. Well there you go, talk about turning lemons into lemonade. It's funny how I will be very happy to find out nowadays if this reaction was made worse by a cold!

Chin up loved ones, I know this has been a long hard slog for you too but we all will get through this. I will now just have to have a "fifty-five and still alive" party instead of a "fifty-four and I ain't knocking on heaven's door" party. I love and adore you and thank you for loving me back.

We are now days from March 2014 and we are still waiting to see what the insurance company comes up with this time. Interestingly enough though, looking back on both of the reports from the two allergists I have seen, even though they have both treated my health differently, I realized that in their reports they do have one thing in common and that is that they both say, "With the onset of Menopause," so it's going to be really interesting to see whether the dermatologists report will say, "with the onset of menopause," or that "menopause doesn't even exist," once we get a copy of it.

I am really tired of fighting for my survival and I am tired of the battlefields, so until I get to "My Healthy and Happy Ending," I think it is time for this:

Dear Medical World,

Wow! What an unnecessary road, health wise, you forced me to travel! As I learnt more about Ms Menopause, I have come to the conclusion she is a bully all because you allowed it! Yep, that's right I am thinking it starts at the top, with you, Medical World. What I have learnt during this journey is that you have put the "secrecy and invisibility" blanket around Ms Menopause by wilfully hiding the truth and facts from women about how big Ms Menopause really is and how debilitating it can be.

I thought about who I am really addressing here, initially it was just the health system, but now it gets directed to the higher powers that be and the bigwigs in the medical world. I am going to direct my anger at the "you" who controls the purse strings and at any "you" who makes the decisions about every woman's health, wellbeing and bloody life during this challenging time.

Fifty to fifty-two, as you are all aware, is the average age women meet Ms Menopause, but women are also meeting her at thirty, forty, fifty and sixty years of age. You have taken it upon yourself to keep the truth from women. Who gave you that right? If a woman was to know the truth and the facts in regard to Ms Menopause and how lots of other factors could come into play that can make a woman's journey with it even more debilitating, then every woman would have more control of this part of their lives and be happier and healthier and be able to retain a sense of who they are.

And stop telling us in your condescending way that menopause is a natural part of a woman's life. We, as intelligent women, bloody well know this! Actually this is the bit about the whole Ms Menopause thing we actually are aware of. Do you think that every time you tell us this, we stand there twirling a strand of our hair around our finger, with our head cocked to one side, chewing gum saying, "Really! Oh my gawd that's, like, so amazing!" It is like you are giving out stupid subliminal messages to control women, so they wander around like zombies who speak like a robot saying, "Menopause is a natural part of a woman's life so we just have to deal with it. Menopause is a natural part of a woman's life, so we just have to deal with it. Menopause is…" well you get the idea.

Now I had to rewrite this whole next paragraph. Initially I could never see the logic in your attitude of, "The less we know the better off we are." The way I saw it, this attitude would put a bigger strain on our health system with all the illnesses and diseases women in this phase of their lives and beyond will deal with. I always thought that if this is your way of thinking, well your thinking is illogical. Today though, with more knowledge, I actually now think it is a deliberate act to keep the pharmaceutical profits up during and beyond our menopause.

Since Ms Menopause knocked on my door, I have never had to visit my doctor so much; I have never had to have so many blood tests and I have never had to take so much medication. I have been admitted to hospital twice for the first time since my daughter was born twenty-two years ago. I have had two trips in ambulances as a patient, I have never had to walk from my job due to ill health before in my whole thirty-six years of working, so that is my strain on the health system, but you know what? That is your doing and your fault! You put this strain on the health system by not giving the truth to woman in regard to Menopause. Now though, I am guessing you are already fully aware of this.

I have had to see two allergists, an endocrinologist, a psychiatrist, a dermatologist who recommended I now see another dermatologist and I have had a visit to a mental health unit. I now see my own doctor more on a regular basis than I see any of my mates. I had to waste precious

279

time to research and find my doctor for BHRT. Oh and imagine the bigger mess I would be in now if I had agreed to everything that your professionals had advised me take in the way of medications.

On top of the steroids, antibiotics, steroid creams plus lots more I have had to live on at times, I would also be taking anti-depressants, sleeping tablets, an immune suppressant drug which is used to stop rejection of organs in transplant patients and HRT. This is the 21st Century, why did my journey have to turn into all this? Well I will tell you why I think this has been allowed to happen. It swings straight back around to the "same old same old," and that is profit, and the dollar is definitely being put before the health of the menopausal woman.

You need to advise women to make a menopausal blood test mandatory, like a pap smear test and a mammogram. Women need to know the tests and options that are out there for them and women need to be able to have these tests in a very easy and simple way. Post-natal depression is a very real thing and is supported by the system. Why is menopause-induced depression not seen as a very real thing and why isn't it supported? Whilst I am here, why would you think that steroids and anti-depressants are the way to care for and deal with menopausal women? It is very clear that you need to have more respect for women who are dealing with Ms Menopause. It is also time that doctors and you too Medical World, are made more accountable for the advice you may see fit to give women.

Oi you! Does this sound disrespectful? Well I hope so as I am now showing you the same lack of respect you have shown me all the way through this. Start the education way back in the classroom. Do you still have those sex education classes that teach the young ones how to have sex? Oops, I mean how to understand their bodies and emotions? Plant the seed then. You teach the girls about their bodies and stages of their lives so why isn't menopause mentioned then as it will be just as much a part, dare I say hugely gigantic part, of their lives as puberty and pregnancy will be. You need to educate women on what will and may happen to many of us, once they are heading into menopause. You are not going to determine when my life is done, that's not your right. This ain't the movie "Logan's Run," y'all!

Now being but one woman, I understand now why your attitude made no sense to me and sounded illogical and ridiculous. It would make sense and there would be less strain on the health care system if women were educated earlier about menopause, but this isn't what you want is it? I have finally grasped the real reason you allow this to be happening to women only now that I am, hopefully, nearing the end of my journey.

You say we are becoming an aging society, so it would make sense to keep menopausal woman healthier so yes, I was confused but also a bit curious as to why all the secrecy around Ms Menopause. I think now though, as I've already mentioned, you help to keep the profits of many pharmaceutical companies high by not telling us the truth. This then ends up with us on all sorts of different medications we will need due to "old age."

I have been advised on two occasions that you feel it is best we menopausal women don't know what can happen to us, but this statement was always ridiculous because that's not the truth. You don't want us to know as we will be healthier and won't have to spend so many dollars which go into the profit margins of the pharmaceutical companies. So who are you? Who are you that you are able to keep our heath system operating in an 1800s mentality regarding menopause? I am also guessing you know the power of the ovary so I can imagine you have a "shoot it down before it can possibly get to it's full potential" attitude.

Wow! There are definitely a few reasons why you would want to keep a good strong woman down when she reaches this stage of her life. We menopausal women help the specialists and doctors to get a good wage each week, we help pharmaceutical companies to keep their profits up by having to be on so much other medication. Oh and just at a time in a woman's life where she is able to, if she wants, climb the corporate ladder and give another good twenty years of her working life. As for me I just wanted to keep earning my dollars for another twenty years, and to be that much needed, healthy and able part of my tribe and live my life in a way I see fit.

Maybe this is your way of dealing with the "growth and decay" theory in our society, or perhaps it is still just a man's world. I don't want it to be a man's world, hell I don't even want it to be a woman's world. I dunno, but I have mentioned to women that "Knowledge is Power". Does this bother you, the fact that women could have the knowledge of what can happen and therefore the power to deal with her earlier and in a way that they choose?

I am not blaming you for the knock on my door from Ms Menopause, which is inevitable in every woman's life. I am not blaming you for my allergies, as Lady Ga Ga would say, "I was born this way." You are not God. I must admit though, I have met a few specialists in my time whilst supporting family, who actually did think they were God but didn't have the God-like attitude. Yes, I did have a chat to one in particular about his bedside manner and attitude and lack of compassion. He doesn't like me much, oh well.

What I do blame you for is not educating me about the fact that Ms Menopause can leave me breathing but feeling I am not alive. I blame you for not educating me about how she can and has exaggerated my existing allergies. I blame you for allowing this natural part of my life to be turned into other illnesses. I blame you for tossing HRT at me and not giving me all my options. I also blame you for not bringing menopause-induced depression into the open...the list just goes on doesn't it?

I don't like the way you have allowed this to affect my earning power, but more importantly I am really, really annoyed at the way you have allowed this to affect my loved ones! Do what you think you can with me, but come near my loved ones and I become a wild beast ready to fight, grabbing on and not letting go and bloody mouthy! Grrrrr!

Also, why the hell have you not informed all women about the link between Ms Menopause and adrenal glands? Now remember I only found this out through my own research, so why are you not telling women about this link? When a woman is suffering so much and they can't function in the world or even in their personal lives, this test should be at least suggested by their doctor. And I am sure there are other links between menopause and the body that I haven't mentioned which make a woman's journey more debilitating than necessary.

Did you know that I have already saved my life twice now? You haven't done this, I have! It's scary to think that you could have allowed my life to end and not even known or given a care. I know one day I am going to pass over, duh, but I want this to be at the end of my natural life, I don't want to, and there is no need to, pass over as a result of Ms Menopause. Even if she does not take a woman's life, she certainly can take away a woman's quality of life. Now, how have I saved my life I hear you say? Well, Of course I am going to tell you.

1. When I was on HRT and I found out, through my own research, that I had to add ten days of progesterone into the mix because I still have my bits intact. If I hadn't found out and only did the HRT gel sachets the lining of my womb could have thickened and caused endometrial cancer! So tell me Medical World, did this turn out to be a man made cancer?

2. When I started dealing with menopause-induced depression and I found out, through my own research, that it wasn't just me. I was really afraid that I was going to buckle under depression and commit suicide. Only finding out the facts gave me the knowledge and power to be able to say, "I am a menopausal woman and I am scared I am going to commit suicide."

Discovering the link between Ms Menopause and our adrenal glands will help some women understand why their struggle with her can be so much more debilitating. With this knowledge in hand it at least gives women a choice of how they can be in control of their own experience.

Why have I had to find all this only through my own research? You should be doing this for all women. When and where, in mainstream society, are the gatherings and the menopause-awareness days? I know you have one now and then, but one now and then is not good enough. Where are the bloody pamphlets? Aren't you in the business of saving lives? What are you getting paid for? I hate to think what could have been if I hadn't looked into Ms Menopause myself and had just gone along with everything you have told me, or if I hadn't found out what you hadn't told me.

I have suffered three-fold throughout my dealings with Ms Menopause. I am dealing with many menopause symptoms. I am dealing with exacerbated allergies, and now I am trying to save myself as you have allowed menopause to turn into an illness. As for A1 and A2, I pray they are only exhausted and not depleted. Once again, this is all your doing. Do you care? Probably not, but I will tell you something now, you are not doing this to my daughter and future generations of women.

I am not angry with my doctor, I am furious with you. Why don't you think it is important enough to even educate doctors properly? Or is it that you have instructed doctors not to tell women all the facts regarding menopause? I am sure the doctor community is answerable to you! This was made pretty damn evident with the pathology nurse who said, "We don't think it is a good idea to bombard women with too much information about Ms Menopause." Now I know who "We" are, it's you!

Each doctor seems to prescribe different ways for women to deal with Ms Menopause as well. I have a friend whose doctor prescribed the pill for her symptoms; she is sixty. I spoke to my doctor to see if this could be an option for me. My doctor was a bit horrified and said no, not a good idea, the pill itself could create other side effects and health issues.

There is nothing uniform in the care of women, it seems at times that doctors are taking pot luck with our health, but again I think it is you putting doctors in this position.

Let us not forget that the basis of menopause is: After a woman's last period, her ovaries make much less estrogen and progesterone. Taking each woman's individual issues, ie allergies and any existing illness or condition out of the equation, can't somebody come up with something that is universal and safe for menopausal women to take to alleviate their suffering?

Well I believe someone has come up with a safe natural option and that is BHRT, that is Bioidentical Hormone Replacement Therapy, Medical World, but you lot still put it down saying it is not scientifically proven. Well have a look at HRT, and you are ok to toss that at us? Oh that's right, we have to keep in mind here the billions of dollars HRT rakes in.

Keep in mind that our existing illnesses and conditions are exaggerated with Ms Menopause, as shown quite clearly by me. If I had been forewarned, even these "side dish" conditions could have been dealt with before they became so debilitating and had caused so much extra suffering. Yeah, you sure have a lot of explaining to do. Actually with what I know now, it would appear that you created all of these allergies in me by not giving me all my options at the beginning, so yeah in my case I would say that all my allergies and everything are definitely a man made mess!

Who gave you the right to decide that you were going to throw millions of women into the "nowhere land" to fend for themselves, who the hell do you think you are? Beautiful women are suffering unnecessarily and are dying too early, and this is your doing. I have read many blogs where women worldwide are searching for answers about Ms Menopause, many having lost faith in their doctors and their health systems due to not being taken seriously, or being told, "It's just menopause."

Hey you! Did you also know that being sick is not cheap? This whole experience has not only affected my earning power, but also the cost of medications and tests etc has added to the financial burden. Here in Australia we have a better health system than many other countries and there is a Health Care card for those who need it, so I do understand we are very fortunate in that respect, but many medications a woman may choose to use during menopause is not covered on this health care card. It only covers what you want it to cover. Hmm there is that controlling us again. We will get our health needs cheaper if we use what YOU want us to use.

Oh, and again YOU stop trying to make out that our health care is a privilege, our heath care is a bloody right! I have paid my taxes, like many other Aussies, for many years. I, like the millions of other Aussies, have proudly contributed to our beautiful country whilst getting on with our lives. You say every Aussie has the right to health care, and yes they do, but they're still being controlled when it comes to the medication they may need.

I want to do my healing and getting my life back naturally. I want to kick Ms Menopause out of the driver's seat of my life naturally, but these options, of course, cost lots of money. I want to live with Ms Menopause peacefully so if I have to put stuff in my body long term, I want it to be natural. I know I could take out private health cover, but I don't want to, I haven't needed it in the past. I did think once that the only way I would do Private Health insurance is if you pay into it and say after 5 years of not needing it, we would get at least a fifty percent rebate back. I say fifty percent approximately as I understand you have to allow for all those administrative costs.

Also throughout my dealings with hospitals through family members, having private health cover doesn't guarantee you won't be sleeping in a ward with public patients, or that you won't have to still wait for that doctor that you want. I have paid for certain health needs privately. We saw the specialist who did my daughter's final operation on her leg privately at times. This wonderful man however, did her operation though the public sector. Every time I have seen my allergist this has been done through the private sector of the health system. I also know that if you are in a private bed and there is an emergency with you needing a private doctor after hours, that you may even be wheeled over to the public hospital ward to be seen by a public hospital doctor.

I also understand the idea that many of you in the medical world might have which would go something like this: "Come on Jen, you are middle aged it is to be expected that you may need private health insurance more as you get older." To a small degree I get that, but my deterioration in my middle age is purely due to Ms Menopause and the fact that you lot didn't educate me or give me the truth about menopause!

Actually what the hell was I paying the Medicare levy at each tax time for? I was still contributing to my own health care. Hey I just had a thought. Do you think maybe you owe me a rebate on all the Medicare Levy I had not used for my health needs until this battle with Ms Menopause began? Actually you keep it because I am using it all now with Ms Menopause knocking, and you not informing me of what I was going to encounter.

Let's also talk about the financial side of all this. As I've already mentioned, due to you not giving women the facts on Ms Menopause, I have had to use money I should not have had to at this age. Are you going to pay that back into where I have to take it out of? It doesn't stop there though. I have lost my earning power, I have lost my superannuation payments paid by my employer, and as of today I have lost sixteen months of these payments into my superannuation fund. I have had to access my saved superannuation twenty odd years before I had planned to so are you going to take responsibility for this? I could have been at my place of employment for over six years now, with only four to go until my ten year long service leave was due. You need to be very aware of the ripple affect Ms Menopause may have on women and their families as well.

Sure, you keep throwing HRT at us, and yes now we know about the side effects that come with it, but let us not forget it's a billion dollar industry. Of course women who are desperate for some sort of relief from their suffering will still use HRT. They know what the side effects are, but what choice have they got? You know that this HRT is a danger to women. Who knows, somewhere, someone could be working on the next better, safer, improved synthetic HRT "thing", but no doubt some time in the future it will probably do the same as those that are thrown at us today.

Ok, STOP PRESS, again. You already knew that natural progesterone is available by script here in Australia that can be prescribed by our doctors, and that there are two natural estrogens already on the PBS, so why the hell haven't we women been given this as a choice by our doctors? You keep tossing HRT at us without giving us any alternatives when you know damn well that there is an alternative to HRT. Why not?

You tell us that the illnesses and symptoms we are experiencing are just a part of old age. You know this is not true! They are preventable fall-out created by Ms Menopause. How can you sit there knowing this and yet say nothing? Are women worth so little that you are willing to compromise their health for profit? And what gives you the right to make the decision to take grandmothers, mothers and daughters away from their families too early and unnecessarily?

What right have you got to withhold all this vital and important information from women? You know menopausal women are screaming out for help all around the world.

Yeah, I believe it's the right time, after so many centuries, that we take back control of our bodies and wellbeing during menopause and demand to be told the truth, demand to be listened to, demand to be believed and demand to be respected.

Menopause was meant to be a celebration of a wonderful time of change in a woman's life, it should be a thank you for everything she has done and will continue to do. We should be able to walk into this next phase of our lives prepared, happy and healthy, but you have taken the celebration out of menopause. Celebrations need preparation, so give women all the truths and information they need to be able to celebrate their menopause instead of drowning and disappearing in it.

I found the following as I was researching and I couldn't agree more:

"The menopausal woman's wisdom is essential for survival, and the more we recognize this truth, the more menopause will be celebrated in our culture."

With no respect,
Jenni

Phew! Glad that's done. That would have to be the biggest mouthful I have ever given anyone in one sitting in my whole life, well except for Sicko Fraud, but I must admit it felt pretty damn good too because they feckin deserve it!

Oh, and since I mentioned Sigmund Freud again I have just found out that his daughter Anna Freud submitted a letter to the Library of Congress in 1952 with instructions that it is not to be opened until 2020. The 2020 would ensure that Anna would have passed over by the time the letter is opened.

I can guarantee this beautiful "child" suffered at the hands of her father and the letter will confirm that Sigmund Freud was nothing but a drugged up paedophile who makes me sick to the core, and this disgusting creep set the foundation for the treatment and attitude towards menopausal women? Yeah I am very saddened that this little girl, Anna, back then had to suffer such abuse at the hands of this sicko, but am looking forward to 2020 to see what truths the letter reveals about Sicko Fraud. What chance did this innocent child have back then? Nada! Ok, in usual style I need to have another shower to clean the disgust and filth off me after talking about Sicko Fraud again, but once that is done it is time to continue the journey.

Chapter 42

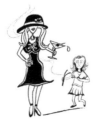

AND ONWARDS WE GO—FEK!

March 2014: Autumn in Australia and it is my favourite season. Not too hot and not too cold, well here in Brisbane it can still feel like summer, but it will cool down. I have always called it my "soul" season, I just love autumn.

Ok, that "self-inflicted" flare up at the end of February actually wasn't self-inflicted and it did turn into a 'flu. Yay! I was sick as a dog for days but this meant that I am travelling ok and that I just caught something. I still have to be careful as I am able to catch bugs easier at the moment because of the way my immune system is, but on the positive side this bug didn't land me in hospital like the bug I caught in 2013. Triple yay!

I went to see my own doctor once I felt a bit better. I also wanted to see him as it has been six months since I had had full blood tests done. I just wanted to ensure Ms Menopause hadn't sneakily thrown anything else into the pot of ills whilst I was concentrating on the day-to-day ills. I also wanted my IGE - allergy rate - checked as it had been sitting at 19500 in September 2013. Normal allergy rate is 0-100. My doctor commented on the fact that my skin wasn't looking as red and inflamed; this was something we at home had also noticed. When the blood test result came back I got a call from the nurse saying my doctor wanted me back in to discuss the results, so an appointment was made.

You know I had all weekend to worry about what he was going to say. I don't know, I thought one only gets called back if all is not looking too good, and my mate tried to reason that maybe he just wanted to discuss the results and that all is ok. I spent that whole weekend thinking about it and the main thing I thought about was cancer. With all that I have dealt with and all that I still deal with I have always been very thankful that the word cancer has never been mentioned. I spoke to the tribe and said with much selfishness that I don't want to have to battle anymore than I have so far. I rocked up for my appointment and the first thing I said to my doctor was, "I don't want the "C" word mentioned!"

He did look at me a little strangely and for that second I thought, "Oh my God he is going to say the "C" word." What he actually said was, "Your results show that your cholesterol is a little high." No wonder he looked at me strangely, cholesterol starts with C, "Your Vitamin D is a little low as well otherwise all shows normal.

Wow! I was so thankful and also a little amused as he seemed to be a bit hesitant in mentioning the "C" word, cholesterol, after my opening announcement. But he left the best part until last. He handed me the results for my IGE - allergy rate - and it showed that in the six months I had been using BHRT my IGE had come down to 9700. Wow! Down from 19500 to 9700! I literally jumped out of my seat. Who was more excited, my doctor or me? We even did a high five together and he congratulated me. Thanks again doc, but I ain't doin' what I am doin' for the kudos, I am doin' it to be healthy, happy and me and for my daughter. Yahoo! My BHRT doctor would be advised as he gets copies of my results, and my allergist who I had cancelled in March and rebooked in May would also be aware as he also does the pathology - the results - for blood tests.

My IGE results came in later than the other results, I was a bit curious as to why, but after getting that wonderful result I can imagine my allergist went, "Huh? I only saw her in September and it was 19500, I've got to check this as now it is 9700! Huh?"

I cancelled my appointment with him in March as I couldn't afford to see him. Even though he has bulked billed me more times than he has charged me, I didn't want to walk in assuming and expecting him to bulk bill me. Also, I haven't needed to see him yet. I could go and see him but it would be a matter of him looking at me and me looking at him and saying nada because as I have said, those drugs he wanted me to go on initially are never going to touch my lips!

So there you go! The best news we have had since 2010. Phone calls were made and sms's and emails were sent to let all know of the results. To be honest that IGE is even lower than the 13000 reading back in 1999 where I found out I was allergic to the dog. So does this now prove that I needed to get my hormones checked after giving birth? I know I still have a long way to go and we are now working on getting my adrenal glands strong and healthy again, and I am still coming off synthetic steroids. I still get tired, my body gets sore and I still don't handle stress, any stress, well, but you know what? I yam what I yam and I yam ecstatic, grateful and just damn happy!

I also gave the draft of my book to a mate to read. It was quite scary handing it over. Besides my immediate loved ones and my best mate, none of my mates know the extent of what I have been dealing with. So yeah, a bit scary but also exciting. I need the draft to be read by someone I trust and this mate is just that.

Before I received those glorious results, I had been back in contact with two mates and let them know in a small way what I had been dealing with. You know it took me until February 2014 to have contact with them but I remember thinking, "Something must be happening with my health as I now have the energy and desire to reconnect with my mates." I am not socializing with them as I did the past, my health and energy are not there yet, but being in contact with them through sms and emails again is a great start.

So to end March I have just gone down to 5mg of steroids. I was able to go down to 6mg and hold for a month, I am still doing BHRT, of course! I now take two low odour garlic tablets instead of the adrenal tablets, a bit of an experiment actually. Yeah, the adrenal tablets were costing me ninety bucks a fortnight for the amount I needed. I could squeeze it to forty-five bucks a fortnight but after reading more about garlic, I thought I would do an experiment. Health is more important than the dollar, I fully understand that, but if I can do it with garlic tablets, which are a hell of a lot cheaper, well that's what I am doing. I've only been doing the garlic for two weeks so the experiment is still in progress.

Garlic is packed full of antioxidants. I always knew garlic was a natural antibiotic but there's more. It helps to strengthen your immune system and is proven to have anti-inflammatory properties. Because it boosts your immune system it helps to improve your adrenal gland's health. Now, the odourless tablet apparently is garlic that has been aged. It is said that the good old smelly garlic is the best, but for me, nah! I do take low odour garlic tablets so we will wait and see.

I am also walking, yep! Got past that three-day fizzle out stage. I had promised myself I was going to start walking on the first day of autumn but didn't. I started on the 11th of March, the day after getting those fabulous results from my doctor. I know walking is good for vitamin D, but apparently it is also good for lowering cholesterol. I have never had a problem with my cholesterol in all my life, I had heard of it, but what is it? Well it is a waxy, fat-like substance that is found in all cells of the body. High cholesterol means you have too much cholesterol - fat - in your blood. Yeah that was enough for me to know that I had to start walking. I started off with fifteen minutes and have built up to thirty to forty minutes a day. I have only now started to attempt some hills.

It is tiresome at times, but not once this time round have I had to ring a loved one to come pick me up due to tiring out. I used to think walking was boring but I had to change my mind-set. Walking gives us a vitamin D hit, helps to strengthen bones to stop osteoporosis, massages and makes adrenal glands happy, that is if they haven't karked it, helps to increase serotonin levels which helps combat menopause induced-depression and helps also to combat menopause-induced insomnia.

Not to mention lowering cholesterol. So much goodness in a walk that will cost you nothing, fabulous! I now walk giving thanks to the universe for my able legs and the fact that the BHRT is a bloody winner! You beauty! My world has just become bigger by thirty to forty minutes on a daily basis.

Oh and did you notice I haven't spoilt all the good news in March by mentioning the insurance company? I will get to the updates in regard to "that mob" in the next few months, for now though I am going to bathe in all my blessings.

April 2014: That feckin insurance company! I don't know when it became acceptable for an insurance company to lie, delay, prolong and just use specialists' material to suit them but more on them shortly.

I am still walking. I have missed a few days but I have had to incorporate walking into my daily life. I say it is another daily medication I need, so I do it. My life is getting a bit bigger with the walking, and I joined our local library that is a five-minute drive away. I don't get there often, but yeah, my life is getting there. I also got one of Dr John Lee's books out from the library; apparently he had written a few. I thought since my own journey with ill health is getting there, it was time to read Dr John Lee's book. The only one they had at the library was *What your doctor may not tell you about Premenopause.* Dr Lee covers a woman's age from thirty to fifty in this book. I am still reading it and I may only be a "girl in the world", but his book confirms for me that my own journey with menopause and my book is on the right track. If you can, grab a copy. His books might seem a lot to take in at times but they are worth reading.

In the last days of April, I was able to go down to 4mg of steroids and I am ok. I still have flare ups but not as constant as before. I still cannot deal with stress, my back aches at times and my energy level is still low. I miss me! I miss that short wild-haired woman who was always able to take life "head on". I want to feel like me again, I want to see me again in my eyes. I want to feel life again. I know I am fighting hard to get old, but I want my happy and healthy ending in this real little life of mine. I want it for me, but mostly I want it for my family.

I feel as if I have already done my old age in my fifties by going through this journey, so, god willing, I will be running amok in my eighties with that sixty year old toy boy by my side! Ah what the heck, I am hoping to be running amok all by myself!

At April 2014 my daily medical needs are: BHRT, synthetic steroids, a walk and water. I still need my steroid cream for my skin on occasion, but that's it! Makes me shiver to think what medication I would be on today and what state my health, physically, mentally and emotionally, would be in if I hadn't researched Ms Menopause.

Chapter 43

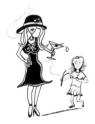

WALKING, CREEPS AND DOGS

Ok, I have already spoken about my walking but I also noticed there is another world out there of walkers and even joggers who whizz past me. The majority of them are a nice lot of people but we don't chat, we just say hi or nod. Who has the breath to chat? When I walk I am concentrating on my breathing and that's about it. Unfortunately, I have met a few who are a bit, well, creepy.

The first one is a nice old bloke I used to say hi to as I passed his house. This bloke would be in his eighties. After a while, even with his walking cane, he started to do a little walk. When I saw him I congratulated him, then he walked over to where I was standing for a second and, no joke, put himself right in my personal space! This made me feel very uncomfortable even before he started to ask where I lived and so on. I know that a lot of elderly people are lonely and I have great respect for them. I am always happy to say hi as it may be the only hello they may get. I did meals on wheels for a while and I have seen the loneliness of the elderly first hand. It was really sad, but I don't like my kindness being seen as a weakness and this bloke really did make me feel uncomfortable, so I told him I had to keep walking and I have found a new walking path. Am I overreacting? Maybe, but I still think there was no need for him to put himself right in my personal space, he could have quickly chatted to me from his side of the road as I was walking past.

The second bloke was around his late fifties and was walking very slowly with a limp. He said hi and me back at him. He then started to tell me about his injured leg. I do listen but I am very aware that I have to keep walking as if I stop I may not start again. Anyhoo I met this bloke a couple of times as I walked and told him I noticed he was walking better, then I just headed on my way. The last time I saw this bloke I had just turned a corner and saw him up ahead. He turned around, saw me and stopped as if he was waiting for me. Yeahnah that ain't gonna happen! So I pretended to be on my phone talking and took a new path. I really don't want to hurt anyone's feelings but I am simply out there to walk to help me get back to me. I don't see walking as a social thing, if anything I have become a little lone wolf throughout this journey. God willing, I will socialize again but I will choose who I allow to be in my personal space.

Now finally, dogs. On a few occasions I have walked right into dogs that are not on a chain. One owner told me that her dog was really friendly. All I could think of saying back was "Oh, ok, rightio." Another woman also told me that her dog was really friendly. This time I asked her to hold her dog as I walked past. People, put your dogs on a feckin leash when out and about! We have a dog that is really friendly, but we also, as much as we love her, understand that she is still a dog. Ours may be old and friendly but we reckon she would still "gum" you to death if you came near any of us, so have consideration for others, there is a dog park a two minute drive from our streets, bloody well go there and let your dog off the feckin chain! Geez almighty!

Yeah, so that's that. Am I now going to fight for the rights of the walker? Nah! I just want to walk safely and by myself without isolating myself as I walk.

Chapter 44

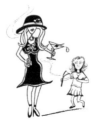

UPDATE ON INSURANCE COMPANIES, AND ONWARDS...

Now a quick update on the insurance company, and yes the following is the short version. Apparently we are now at their "procedural fairness" stage. Ha ha he he chuckle chuckle, oops sorry it is all so laughable. Ok, do you remember that first allergist who was put out to pasture regarding my claim? Well the insurance company have decided that now his material is "satisfactory". Do you remember that "shrink" I saw in 2013? Well I found out that he put my depression down to losing my sister in 2004 and the insurance company plucked his report out of all the others from 2013. Yep, this is all material the dermatologist, who I had to see in January or pay 1000 buttons, got to work with, including my doctor's consultations and blood test results. Actually the insurance company didn't even give the dermatologist a copy of the material from the first allergist and only gave him material that ended in March 2013. Go figure eh?

So he was only given copies of my doctor's consultations, blood test results and the shrink's report. They omitted my second allergist and my BHRT doctor, everything from March 2013 up to today, April 2014. I do wonder, is that even legally allowed?

It is too long and drawn out to talk about it all, but my lawyer is onto it. On the positive side though, the dermatologist did feel that my problems stemmed from menopause, yahoo! So we are still dealing with "that mob" and I will update the outcome, hopefully, before the end. Two things I will say are: "Oi, Insurance Company, I ain't seeing any procedural fairness towards me in regard to my claim," and, "Oi Shrink, I found your assessment of me disrespectful. How dare you insult my daughter by writing that I was trying to snuff myself out due to losing my beautiful sister nearly ten years ago! My daughter has been the main reason I want to live throughout this journey with Ms Menopause, so pull your 'expert' head in. It still gob-smacks me to think that you were prepared to stick me on anti-depressants because of your incorrect assumption about me losing my sister. I know I sat there giving you answers to your questions but how dare you even mention my beautiful sister in regard to my menopause! Just grasping at straws weren't you? Lucky I didn't mention I had lost my first love in a bike accident when I was twenty-one, as no doubt you would have 'conjured' that up as a reason for my mental state as well. I don't know whether to be really angry with you or just laugh at you due to the ridiculousness of your 'expert' assessment of me. The first word that comes to mind when I think of you is 'twit!' God help all of your other patients."

I sit here and wonder, who are these experts that we have to deal with? In a land a long time ago before Ms Menopause knocked at my door, I only dealt with specialists on behalf of others. Since I have had to deal with them for myself, it scares me to think that we put our faith in them, and at times they think they can say and do whatever they see fit. To be fair though, I am only talking about some of the "experts" I have dealt with and I know I have come up against it because of the word "menopause".

May 2014: Well the cold snap came…brrrrrrrr! And went! I got down to 4mg of synthetic steroids this month and am holding. I have gone back on my adrenal tablets but am finding that my back is constantly sore even with them. I have noticed my energy levels are lower and it's a bit push and shove just to stay awake for a whole day, but my skin hasn't flared up as much as I was expecting. I haven't been down to 4mg of synthetic steroids for a very long time, so I actually wasn't sure what was going to happen. I am still walking, am missing days here and there but mostly I walk. I find when I do have a flare up I feel more swollen, but still walk as much as I can. I really want to walk every day, so hopefully that is coming.

May has been a bittersweet month. Eurovision is on! Yay! And the final fell on Mother's Day! Double yay! It is also the month of the ten-year anniversary since we lost my sister to leukaemia. Yeah, even though I keep her in my heart every day, it seems forever since she was here. I love you Helen. I know as I write I feel flat and reading back on May I'm aware of this feeling coming through, but I am still getting there and am still in a better place since I put myself in the driver's seat with my health. I think I expect too much too soon as I was so healthy before menopause.

Funnily enough I kept coming across the expression "You can't hit the ground running!" over the period of a few days. Then it hit me, how true. I guess I was expecting to hit the ground running, but even though I get impatient to get "there" with my health, it is still going to take time and that, I have learnt, is just something I have to accept. Hearing and seeing that saying wasn't just a coincidence. I really was getting quite despondent over all this, so I reckon it was my family putting it all into perspective for me. Yes you are all right, I can't hit the ground running, well not yet anyway. This, God willing, is my healing period so I have to be patient. Thanks loved ones, I love you all!

I still cannot deal with stress. I still have backache, bloating, and at times inflammation and swelling. On occasion my skin is red but only in sections of my face, but on the positive the hair is back! Huh? Yep my hair has come out of the ponytail. Throughout this journey with Ms Menopause my hair was always put up in a ponytail. For some reason, as much as I am very thankful for my hair, it annoyed me. So yep the hair is back, a bit blonder… oh ok, a bit greyer, but it's out doing its thing again.

Am I functioning better on a day-to-day basis? Well yes I am. To compare my day with how I was before this journey, no I am not functioning as I used to, but I am definitely functioning better since I started my BHRT. I am hoping A1 and A2 kick back in and I think they already are, but only time will tell. Am I feeling more fatigued now due to coming off steroids after depending on them for so long? Yes. Am I feeling more fatigued due to A1 and A2 having to do their thing again without the aid of the synthetic steroids? Yes. So I am getting there. Regardless of how much longer this all may take I know I am on the good side of it now, for me the only way is upwards and onwards, it may be slow and steady, but I'm looking forward to finally feeling like me again.

June 2014: Winter in Australia. June actually started off as a good month. In June I was able to get down to 3mg of steroids and I can tell you I have not been able to get that low since 2011.

My walking continues, I even did a hill that I had been eyeing off for a while and I can tell you now when I got to the top of that hill huffing and puffing I wished I had a "Meno" flag to plunge into the ground when I hit the top! It felt good to know that I had finally conquered this hill.

I started walking again in March and I keep a diary of my efforts and noticed that each month I am walking more days than the previous month. I have gone back to the garlic tablets and have stayed on them. I noticed that even on the adrenal tablets I was still experiencing everything still so yeah, back on the garlic tablets for good now.

I felt for a while that this was now becoming "The evolution of the menopausal woman." Seriously. My walking has gone from my knuckles dragging on the ground, with a not-so-straight spine as I grunted and huffed and puffed over all the streets I walked, to being able to walk a bit faster with a straight back, to doing a few hills. I also went from announcing every morning, "I really don't want to walk but I have to," to "I'm doing my walk now," to actually looking forward to my walk. I really felt that I had become a true blue walker.

Unfortunately, June didn't end as well as it started. I woke up one morning mid June feeling dizzy. This stopped and I went for my walk. Five days later I woke up with my left eye puffy, a bit red, and my back was sorer than normal. This continued for the next five days with both eyes starting to swell, but I still walked. In the wee hours of the next morning I woke up having problems breathing, but that settled down. I then woke up with my chest congested and a cold, feeling like death on legs! Feck!

I was really doing well then had to catch this on top of it all. I had to stop walking at the end of June as I was too sick. This infection started mid June and continued into July. I booked an appointment with my doctor early July and I know I still have to be aware of my immune system, but I was doing really well, so knew something else must be happening. I don't know how I came upon it, but I read somewhere that tapering off long term synthetic steroids brings other side effects. Feckin fabulous! I know I have to come of the steroids slowly for my safety and I know that I am going to feel more fatigued as a result, but you know not one bastard thought to advise me that there would be other side effects in doing this! Anyway, I will discuss it all with my doctor in July when I see him.

I will say though that I reckon A1 and A2 are waking up. I may struggle a bit more getting off the last of these steroids, but I am still on a lower dosage than I have ever been on throughout this journey. Come on A1 and A2, you can do it! We have come this far and I know the battle continues, but we've got to be able to get off these feckin synthetic steroids!

July 2014: Brrrrrr! It's been a bit so chilly here in Brisbane. Apparently we had our coldest morning since 1911. Freezing! I am now down to 2mg of steroids and I crawled into July as I still am not well. I see my doctor on the 9th to get a check up. I have noticed my mood seems to be dropping again, not full on depression, but yeah, I just feel down. I initially thought that it may be due to being despondent after doing so well then getting sick, but after investigation I found there are so many side effects to tapering of steroids, even when doing it slowly to give A1 and A2 a chance to produce their own natural steroids again with the help of BHRT.

Tapering off steroids not only causes fatigue, it also can weaken your immune system which in turn makes it easier to get infections. Look at me! And besides another list of side effects it can also cause depression. Ah ha! Look at me again. Ok! Rightio, so now I am dealing with getting off these steroids. Knowledge is power, and now knowing these facts, I am hoping this is what is affecting me so badly.

So I could feel my mood dropping, but this time I spoke to my loved ones about it. It was a bit hard because I don't want them to worry, but I had to let them know that the depression I was starting to feel again was just being caused by the steroids. I did tell them that it didn't feel as big as it was before, but I was just making them aware.

On the day of seeing my doctor he checked my blood pressure which was fine, but my heartbeat apparently was too fast. He asked me if I had been feeling dizzy. Gulp! Um yeah, but only once back in mid June doc. He then got me attached to an ECG just to check my heart, but all was ok. I told him that I had been suffering with this infection since mid June and he said that I should have come and seen him sooner as he would have not let me go down to 2 mg of steroids. You know when he said this I could feel my nose screw up like that Scottish kid on that old commercial when he is given yucky porridge and says, " Tha no how you make porridge!" in a thick Scottish accent. Except my nose was screwed up saying, "But I really want to get off these steroids." In an Aussie accent!

Before finding out about the hazards of tapering off steroids and before chatting to my doctor, not once did I think this chest infection had anything to do with lowering the amount of steroids I am on. I know I should have seen my wonderful doctor earlier but just having the energy to get to him is sometimes really hard. I know I was walking and getting out of the house, but there is no preparing for that. That is just a matter of getting up, getting changed, eating to be able to take my medication, then out the door. It doesn't matter if my hair is not brushed as it gets thrown into a ponytail, it doesn't matter if I am not showered as I am just walking on my own. Getting prepared to see my medical people is such a different and bigger event.

We also had a good chat about the side effects and symptoms of the tapering time. I walked out of there feeling a bit better knowing that all I may have to deal with in the coming months and beyond may be exaggerated due to getting off these feckin steroids. I know it sounds scary, but as long as I am educated and have knowledge, I will be able to deal with it all a bit better. So for me, no! I haven't taken lots of steps backwards, yes the BHRT is still doing its job, yes A1 and A2 are coming back to life, I just have to get through this tapering off steroids phase.

When I got the chest infection I also lost all interest in walking, who doesn't when they are sick, but my enjoying walking went from enjoyable right to have no bloody interest in it anymore and I just don't feckin want to work hard for my health anymore if it ain't gonna happen! But I understand now that I am still getting there, I've just got to adjust to the tapering off phase. I now want to start walking again, so hopefully soon.

You know I can't wait until all I am on is my BHRT, garlic tablets and my A1 and A2 are healthy again. I still don't know exactly how I will feel once I can take what I want without synthetic steroids being in the mix. I was a bit scared to go down to 1mg at the end of July so I only went down to 1.5mg of the synthetic steroids. But as you will see in August, my saying went from "some days are diamonds, some days are stone," to "some days are stone, some days are pebbles," to "some days are pebbles and most days are becoming rubble!"

Before we head into August, I look back on this journey and realise I have been offered to have three bits of me chopped off! My doctor wanted to get rid of a thing on my neck, but I said no! He advised me what to watch out for if it was anything ugly, but so far so good. My BHRT doctor wanted to do a biopsy on the discolouration of my skin, but I said no! I don't want a bloody stitch! The third offer was after I was admitted to hospital in 2012. I read that they had said that perhaps a bowl biopsy could be done. I didn't have to say no on that one as that was the first of that request I had heard of. Wow! Maybe we are not much different to the menopausal women of the past who had bits of them chopped off by moronic medical men. The difference today is the bits they want to chop away at and the fact that women have more of a voice nowadays. Bloody scary though!

And have you noticed that Ms Menopause has not been mentioned for a while? Yep, she is an artiste. She came and took over my life in 2010 but here I am today dealing with symptoms from tailoring off synthetic steroids which I was put on in 2011 due to her, but, it appears that she is nowhere to been seen. Never forget that all I have dealt with and continue to deal with is all of MS Menopauses doing regardless of how far away from her it seems.

Chapter 45

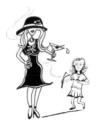

HAPPY NEW YEAR 2015!

January 2015: Huh? I hear you all thinking, "What happened from August up to December?" Yeah well about that… I haven't been able to write since July 2014. That chest infection/flu/whatever that started in June continued right up to September 2014. Another reason I haven't been able to write is the fact that we lost our beautiful old dog Ginger in August 2014.

I know being sick stops me from writing at times but when we lost Ginger, which was so sad and heartbreaking, I lost all desire to write. I know people may say she was only a dog, but to me she was family. We had her for sixteen years so when she passed not only did we grieve for our beautiful old girl, but for me it also flung me back sixteen years to the memory of my daughter being in Grade One when we brought Ginger home. It also brought out my inner child where at times the thought of not seeing her again made me want to sob, demanding, "I want to see Ginger and I want to see her now!" Vale Ginger! Like all our family that has gone before us, I will miss you forever. Thank you for all your love and loyalty. I have visions of you with Pop, playing ball as you both used to do in the backyard. Oh and yes, I am very relieved to know I am not going crazy when I have felt your paw on my heel as I walk, something you would do when you wanted to play, as other family have also felt it. I know you still watch out for us, and with all due respect, we also know you are around as we can smell you quite strongly at times, so that last bath that you fought so hard against and which because of your age you won, may have not been such a bad idea after all. Love you Ging, will miss you forever, just ensure you are bathed by the time we meet up again my beautiful friend.

August 2014: I was taken to hospital by ambulance due to splattering and to the fact that my blood sugar levels were very low. A week later, we lost Ginger. So I just kept crawling through August, and had to up my steroids for three days back up to 12mg, then back down to 6mg where the whole ordeal of trying to taper off these bloody things re-starts. This month also saw me saying goodbye to my lawyer who had been handling my insurance claim.

Firstly, I am still always grateful to my lawyer for taking this on for me in February 2012, but in hindsight and knowing what I know now, I should have shopped around for a firm that has expertise in insurance claims. I just thought all lawyers knew it all but they don't, they have expertise in different sections of the law. When I could see that the insurance company was acting in bad faith over my claim but were not being made responsible for their actions, and when my case was handed to a third lawyer in this firm who seemed like he couldn't give a rats backside, well that was enough for me to call it quits with that firm. I have been fighting for my health for many years now. I don't need a lawyer who is not prepared to fight for my rights with my insurance claim.

September 2014: It was only in mid-September that I woke up feeling like I was over the ill health that I had been dealing with since June. I now felt like I was back to just dealing with my everyday ill health. So it took from June to September to get through that extra crap I had to deal with. September also saw me dealing head on with the insurance company. I had sent them a long list of questions that I wanted answered in regard to the way they have dealt with my claim. I did get a response which mostly was pointing the finger at others, but at least they did admit to being at fault in omitting relevant information in regard to my claim, or in their words, an oversight. Will this matter? I don't know, only time will tell.

October 2014: Still just hanging in and tapering off steroids. I look back on a few of these months and realise I was just going through the motion of getting up every day. I know dealing with that crap from June to September knocked me out, but losing our beautiful old dog in amongst it really made me feel like "why bother, it's all too feckin hard". I know now that a lot of grief was thrown into the pot at this time. Even so, I know I have always been a strong little soldier throughout my life, but Ms Menopause really has tested my strength.

I also had blood tests done with my doctor. Unfortunately my IGE rate has risen a bit, but the most surprising thing is that my progesterone level has gone down. I was a bit taken aback at this as I am still on BHRT, so again something else is happening. My only clue, and I need to chat to my doctor about this, is that my oestrogen is a little lower as well. As we all know now, we lose about sixty percent of our oestrogen during menopause and this can take a few years to reach base line, so is the fact that I am losing a bit more oestrogen, which makes my adrenal glands steal from my progesterone, the reason why my progesterone level has come back lower? It really is like sifting through a labyrinth. Until I can get to see my BHRT doctor again I made the decision to up my BHRT, so we will see what happens.

November 2014: Still just hanging in and tapering off steroids. Another month of just going through the motion of getting up every day. I know, I know, I need to count my blessings. I am still here, I am still getting up every day and I still have wonderful family supporting me.

This month I headed off to the dentist to see if I could start work on my teeth after having been told some time ago that I couldn't have any work done on my teeth until I was taking less than 7mg of steroids. Well I was sitting on 4mg now, so off I went.

The dentist was lovely but wasn't prepared to do any work on my teeth until I spoke to my doctor, as he was concerned I might go into adrenal crisis… fabulous! This would mean that I would have to, once again, up my steroids before any extractions could be done. Oh well, it put it all into perspective for me, walk around with my front tooth missing looking like a hobo or have my smile back which might make my adrenal glands go into crisis… hmmm, let me think for a moment… yeahnah. I will keep the hobo look for now. Some have said it looks cute. I say they are only being kind. I couldn't bear to think that A1 and A2 would be in crisis and I have no intention of upping my steroids just to fit nicely in with society again. We will see what 2015 brings.

Chapter 46

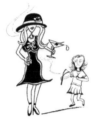

INSURANCE ZZZZZZZ

I also continued to deal with the insurance company. I was able to arrange, at their cost, an appointment with my immunologist in December. I was looking forward to this as I really needed to chat to him, but never are his meds going to touch my lips. I wanted to see him to get those in-depth blood tests done to see how my T cells etc are travelling. The insurance company wanted a report of my updated prognosis as well, but as per usual they threw a spanner in the works.

When I was sent the information regarding my appointment they also sent paperwork that stated that my… *my* immunologist would not be in a treating role at this appointment and that he was only to do a report for the insurance company. Really! You reckon? So I shot them off an email stating that he was to be treating me as his patient at this appointment, that he will continue to be my treating immunologist in the future, that he is fully aware that he will be treating me as his patient at this appointment and in the future, and that I want them to reply in writing in an email that this is how it is to be. And so they did. Of course it came with really cringe-worthy excuses, but I didn't care,

I have now what I need in writing from them. I had to get it in writing as I have learnt that once a specialist does a report for the insurance company they cannot be your treating doctor in the future.

December 2014: Ok, Christmas tree went up and pressies are under the tree. I am happy to just "be" and to share another Christmas with my loved ones. Through facebook, I also re-connected with a few people I had lost sight of while dealing with all this stuff. Yes facebook. I know I said earlier that I don't do facebook, but it's nice to re-connect with a few. My only sadness with it is that I became friends again with a guy I had known who moved to America many moons ago who is now dealing with stage four cancer. That was a real shock. All I could do is throw a huge prayer up to the universe for him. I know illness does not pick and choose, but he is such a beautiful person with such a beautiful heart and soul. I know it's been many moons since we were together but I have no doubt he is just as giving and loving as he was back then; it just seems so unfair!

I also rang my immunologist's office in early December to ensure the appointment had been made by the insurance company, I don't trust that mob! I also rang again after being assured by the insurance company that my immunologist was fully aware that he was to treat me as his patient at this appointment. I spoke to a nice young bloke who assured me that regardless of what the insurance company requested, my immunologist would indeed be treating me as his patient. Ok I thought, good man.

On the 23rd of December 2014 I headed off to see my immunologist. After the "Hi's how yar beens" we sat down to business. I had decided to take the tablet with me to show him photos of my skin since I had last seen him, and after what he said I was so happy I did. Once we sat down he explained to me what the insurance company was requesting of him in his report. He stated that he would not be treating me today as a patient as per the insurance company's instructions. "Oh yes you

313

are!" I retorted, "I have had this out with the insurance company and I have an email from them confirming this." Thank God I took the tablet! He was able to get a copy of the email from the insurance company from my email account and as soon as he read it, off we went, my immunologist and me. So much for that assurance that regardless of whatever, I was his patient! Geez almighty!

As my immunologist was typing something into his computer I looked at the paper work that was on his desk. I saw one sheet had my name on it but...! All I could do was tap my finger on it and say, "That's not me!" Yep, the same issue I had a year ago...the wrong Jenni Townsend's personal details. Again, thank God I noticed that! I don't normally touch paperwork on a medical person's desk but this time I did and saw that! I explained to him what had happened previously, but he hadn't been made aware of this rather important mix-up! Yeah I am damn sure the maker of this error forgot to tell him about it. He apologized and said that it had been coded incorrectly and fixed it up again. My issue though is that my clinical records were still sitting under the other Jenni Townsend's name. Why hadn't this been corrected a year ago? It makes me shiver that this sort of error can happen. As mentioned, this isn't just a pizza order mix-up, this is two people who are fighting for their lives, or I assume the other Jenni is. Well if she wasn't before she could be now due to being on the incorrect medications for her illness. It's just all kinds of feckin wrong!

The rest of the appointment went well. Blood pressure checked, eyes checked for cataracts, none thank god. Yes long-term steroids can also cause cataracts. Spleen touched up a bit and checked. I walked into this appointment struggling on 3.5mg of steroids. I walked out on the advice that I need to go back up to 5mg and come back down monthly by 0.5mg. Going down 1mg a month was too much for me and my body wasn't coping with it. I had gone down 0.5mg for about a month but he wanted me to up my steroids and then come down by 0.5mgs over a longer period. I keep thinking that there is a method in this even though it sounds like "huh?" He also wants to look at putting me on a faster acting blah blah steroid, but we are going to sort this out next time I see him.

I was in with him for over an hour and then had to go off and get six vials of blood done. It was just before I walked out of the appointment that we had a bit more of a chat about the steroids. Long-term steroid use is dangerous, it can affect so much of your body and this is when I started sobbing! I am a menopausal woman in the 21st Century and this nightmare has now been turned into a fight against these bloody steroids. It just keeps getting better. He gave me a tissue and offered me a glass of water but what I really wanted was my family doctor's jar of jellybeans… they always made me feel a bit better after a cry!

When heading home I kept thinking of one of the questions he had asked me which was, "Why didn't you just try HRT?" I explained to him quickly that I had and how it affected me, and how I still shiver today thinking about it. Yeah I kept thinking about this question and I think it was the word "just" that made me think that I should have asked him back, "Why don't you go and "just" try rubbing poison into your body and see how you feel in a wee bit. Bet you ain't gonna feel on top of the world!"

I know he meant no disrespect with this question and I know it wasn't meant to sound flippant, but the "just" made me think, "Don't you know the dangers of HRT to a woman?" I guess it was asked in such a way that it clearly was expected of me to try HRT. Why? Oh and if you are reading this my immunologist, I mean no disrespect, I "just" don't believe that women should feel as if they haven't done everything possible for their health "just" because they choose not to touch HRT with a ten foot pole. Now, with knowledge in hand, I am trying to get my mojo back naturally and safely.

Christmas Day was lovely, although the daughter was a bit sick on the day but is ok now. So I say, doing double shifts is to be admired, but trying to also live the life of a twenty-two year old at the same time, well your body is going to crash and burn, but what do I know my daughter! I will tell you daughter what I know. I didn't get to fifty-four not knowing stuff. So when I say, "Your health is your best asset, I mean it daughter, without your health you'll not be able to make the money you want. Love you, yar mamma! Mwah!"

It was also our first Christmas in sixteen years without our beautiful old dog, so that sat with us a bit as well. I am still very thankful though that you didn't pass over last Christmas day Ginger. My birthday four days later was really lovely too, I was very spoilt. Oh and a quick message to Ms Menopause: these kilos I have piled on over Christmas and my birthday are all my doing and nothing to do with you! Yeah Ms Menopause, I added those kilos on all by myself without any input from you, so suck on that Ms Menopause! You know in another time, another age, I would not be declaring that so proudly. Ha ha hmm.

Oh and how could I forget? My year of being left alone by Centrelink was up in September last year, so they're very, very, very quick to make appointments with me again. I am surprised that one minute after the year was up, they didn't come and drag me out of my bed marching me into their office in my pj's. No joke! I wonder if they employ a person to just sit with their finger hovering over the "your time is up" button counting down the seconds before it can be pushed. I dunno, just saying.

So I submitted a new three-month certificate from my doctor stating I still cannot work as I am still on the Newstart Allowance. I then received notification that I was to attend a five-minute face-to-face chat. I headed down and chatted to one of them. This woman gave me a disability form to be filled out by my doctor. I also had a chat to her about the menopausal woman's plight. Yeah I thought, considering I decided I want to be the voice that stands up for the menopausal woman who is suffering I thought now was as good a time as any. I stood there not giving a crap about who was listening and stated that there is no place in society for the menopausal woman who is suffering. I also said Centrelink hasn't even a place for us.

A bit more was said and you know I felt good in saying it. Will it make a difference? I don't know, but I stood up for me and for others who may be suffering, and even though it was short and sweet, I haven't heard that voice from me for a very long time! I didn't even care if those around me thought I was just a crazy, middle-aged, menopausal woman "having a go", because you know what? Once again they wouldn't be far from the truth! Actually I was more concerned about the big burly security guard who I could see was edging his way slowly towards me. Really?

I was also advised that the time frame for my time out from being hassled and hounded by them and employment agencies actually went for two years. Hmm, ok I thought, so why am I here talking to you Centrelink? After getting this form back from my doctor I headed down to submit it as requested.

I really wasn't feeling too well when I did this. I had just had blood tests done. I was feeling quite groggy and just felt like crap. As it takes all my might to just get ready to see my doctor, I thought that while I was showered, dressed and with all knots extracted from my hair, I would head down to Centrelink to submit this form. I also wanted to get the form in sooner rather than later as I actually thought after all this time sense had arrived and I was going to be put on the disability pension.

You know I really dislike the insurance company. I know, a bit out of context with what I am writing about now, but if it weren't for them messing me around I would have my own dollars. Yes Insurance Company, those dollars are my dollars. You know it, I know and soon the whole world will know it. If you had done your job professionally I wouldn't have had to go in cooee of a Centrelink office. I really dislike your guts! Yeah! Said with much conviction and immaturity! I really want to use the word hate, but it is such a strong word, so dislike it is.

I was originally advised I would only need to pop the form in. I strolled in, explained to the bloke who meets and greets that I just had to hand this form back in. After he brought my customer number up on his tablet he advised me that it might be best if I wait and have a face to face, as they are not too sure what to do with me. Yep! Am I surprised? Nah! All I could say was, "I am really tired will I have to wait long?" Fortunately, he actually listened to me and after taking a seat for a few minutes my name was called out.

I handed this bloke the disability form explaining that I was advised to pop it back in. This what happened next:

Him: What is the point of this form? (Seriously this is what he said! Well for a split second I just looked at him).

Me: I tell you what, you go and ask the girl who advised me to get my doctor to fill this form out and ask her what the point of this form is! You sit there asking me what the point of this form is? It was an employee of Centrelink that gave it to me to fill out so you go ask her what the point of this form is!

Yeah, I was ripe for the taking! I was not only speaking with my mouth but my hands got into it as well, waving all over the place. I wasn't rude, my voice was a little bit louder but I still stated my case respectfully. You know I really can't deal with stress. In the old days before Ms Menopause knocked on my door I was never backward in coming forward, I always stood up against bullying and the way people are treated, but in the end I knew getting upset with this twit wasn't worth the effort or the toll it takes on my health so I just said, "I am not well enough to get upset with you."

The end result was that he didn't accept the form and he booked me in for an appointment with a disability employment agency. So I just let it all go down and walked out knowing I was ringing Centrelink when I got home. And so I did. On the phone I explained what had happened, then was informed that the form I had been given was just part of the process of applying for the disability pension. Oh, ok then. I told her that I felt bullied into having to go to the Disability Employment agency. When she checked my file she advised me that no, I didn't have to attend this appointment as I had submitted a certificate from my doctor stating I could not work. Ok, so why all the bother with the other twit?

The voice on the phone also advised me that I can't stay on Newstart forever and going to the Disability Employment agency moves me to the next phase. You know I loved the way she said, "You can't stay on Newstart forever," like it was my choice. What a joke! Thinking about it later I should have said: "Don't make it sound like it has been my choice to stay on Newstart! I have been enquiring about the disability pension for ages now with no useful feedback or direction from Centrelink. The reason I am still on Newstart is because your office does not know what to do with me!" I am now exhausted. We did agree that I would attend an appointment with the disability employment agency once the doctor's three month certificate expired, which put it to the 22nd of December 2014.

I agreed to this after it was explained to me that I wouldn't be pushed back into work, that I needed to be moved to this next step, and that they are gentler than those other employment agencies. After agreeing to this I thought, "I have a doctor who says I cannot work, I have an immunologist who says I cannot work, I have always been a worker and I know I cannot work," but when I sat down and thought about it, I decided it may be a positive, so we will see when I rock up for it. After getting off the phone I realised this appointment had been set for the day before my immunologist's appointment and this just stressed me to the max! I have a hard enough time getting to one appointment let alone two in a two-day span, but thought I've just got to do it.

We are still working with one car between three of us and I realised the time of this appointment would throw a spanner in the works trying to get the tribe to work, so I rang the agency to see if I could get an earlier appointment. I was advised that I couldn't as they had no times available for that day, I was then advised that I could come in the next day but I had to say no as I was seeing my immunologist. Then they said "if it was ok with me" could the appointment wait until the 5th January 2015? You know what I did? I cried through the phone, yep, just like a big girl's blouse. I explained to her quickly that I can't deal with much at one time and that the new appointment date was perfect. I was so thankful that I didn't have to deal with this one day before seeing my immunologist. Honestly, it's just too feckin stressful.

So here we are in 2015. I have been reading over this chapter and realized that if I had the copyright and wouldn't get sued, I should be calling this chapter "The Never Ending Story" because that is what this journey with Ms Menopause is starting to feel like. I also had a thought. "Do I continue to blame Ms Menopause or is it time to cut her some slack and shift all of the blame onto the medical community?" I have known the answer to this all the way through this book, but it's the first time I actually asked myself this question. OMG, as Ms Menopause has been in my life for so long am I starting to feel sorry for her. Geez Jenni, she ain't even a real person!

But imagine for a moment she is a real woman. Then imagine Ms Menopause is you. It is your profession to knock at every woman's door at this time in her life. You are very good at what you do, you know your stuff and you are very professional, well you have been doing this job for centuries so yeah, you are at the top of the food chain in your profession. Now imagine that you are dismissed and ignored by the medical community and society in general and anyone that meets you has such a dismissive attitude towards you and won't believe what you are really capable of, well yeah! I would feel sorry for you, oh I mean her, too. So I say to you Ms Menopause, I apologise for calling you a "bitch", actually it was three times, when I was whinging about you to some mates. I also say to self: "Get a handle Jen, she ain't a real person!"

When a person is diabetic, they are treated for that illness. When a person is asthmatic, they are treated for that illness. When a person has cancer, they are treated for that illness. When a person has a mental disorder, they are treated for that illness. When a woman is losing hormones due to menopause why is this not taken seriously? Sure menopause is a natural part of a woman's life, but the illnesses women live with as a result of losing these hormones does, as far as I am concerned, open up a gigantic can of worms when we ask who is really responsible for all the ills and medical mistreatment a woman may face at this time.

Well the answer is: The majority of the medical world, the pharmaceutical companies who are only interested in dollars, society in general to a degree, and lastly, we women who have to take some responsibility for it. We are menopausal women in the 21st Century. We need to stand up and say loudly "Not good enough!" We need to talk about it and instead of it being a "taboo" subject we need to get it out into the open. Let us never forget that HRT is killing women. Ok off me invisible soapbox once again.

So it's time to soldier on into a New Year and honestly the thought of it exhausts me again. I have been back on 5mg of steroids for just over two weeks and I am bloody tired. I am having moments of wanting to sleep more again so I fight against it to get through a full day awake and conscious. Before I knew it I was heading into the appointment with the disability employment agency. I was still quite stressed about going. I guess my greatest fear is that I am going to be pushed into doing something that I know I am not capable of. I didn't really know what to expect when I got there. To be honest I was expecting people in wheelchairs and that I would be the only able bodied person there with all my limbs. I know disability comes in all different forms, but many disabilities are not so obvious at times, and I thought I would have another fight on my hands having to prove my illness.

The appointment went well. I was asked why I had been sent there. I explained and also said that they had admitted that they didn't know what to do with me. The interviewer just shook her head with a "yeah that's Centrelink for you" look. The interviewer asked why I hadn't been put on Disability payments. Before I answered I rolled my eyes and she said, "Ok so that is also another story about Centrelink?" All I could say was yep, I told her a bit about the saga and she was quite disgusted at how I have been treated by Centrelink.

We went through everything and she was wonderful! The interviewer could see that I wasn't well and she agreed to let me have more time to just work on my health. I wasn't being pushed into work, thank God! I don't know what would have happened if I was. Actually, yes I do. I can't work. Out of all the doctors, specialists and organisations involved with my health situation, Centrelink is the only one who thinks I can. I would have had to say "No I can't," which would have put a stop to my payment. I dislike you heaps insurance company!

The Interviewer and I chatted for over an hour and it was a really nice atmosphere. I walked out of there feeling like the weight on my shoulders had lifted a bit. I go back in just over two weeks, but now I know what to expect I am actually quite looking forward to it!

It is now early January 2015. I am now waiting to hear from the insurance company as they would have received my immunologist's report by now. I also have to see my doctor soon to get a few checks done and get some more results back. . I just want everything to fall into place this year. First health and then finances.

Chapter 47

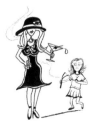

FEBRUARY 2015 ONWARDS

February 2015: Firstly, the comment I made in January about how the insurance company would have received my immunologist's report was just wishful thinking on my part. Ok, I heard nothing in regard to my claim in January. On the 6th of February 2015 I received a letter from my superannuation fund advising me that they were still waiting to receive the report from my immunologist and when they asked for a timeframe for completion the receptionist told them, "Eight weeks as the doctor is very busy." So now it is just over six weeks since the appointment I attended on the 23rd of December 2014 and we have been advised it will take another eight weeks for the insurance company to receive this report? So it's going to take fourteen weeks! So, here we go again I thought, more delays and problems, but this time I can't blame the insurance company. The only thing I am curious about is why the insurance company took six weeks to follow it up. February was a pretty tough month, but I am guessing it's like that for many households when bills come in, so concentrating on that, I didn't put much effort into chasing the report, but why should I? Isn't that supposed to be the insurance company's job?

February saw the normal bills - rates, electricity and water - come in. It also saw the renewal of the registration for the one car we still have. It also saw this one car we still have decide to take a turn for the worse, and it had to be towed up to our mechanic. Yep! Right in the middle of all the other stuff that had to be paid out. Fabulous. Now I have not been able to work since July 2012, yes I am getting the Newstart allowance, but the combined family funds are starting to look a wee bit non-existent. This is when I decided not to get my new lot of BHRT so that I could help with all the other bills that needed to be paid. You know my tribe doesn't even know I did this, they would have been horrified, but I was feeling a bit selfish spending money on the BHRT when I knew it could help with household and car costs. So I stopped it. Now daughter when you read this in say twenty odd years, no point bringing up the past now, ok?

I have continued to have appointments with that employment agency and am feeling pretty good about it. Now let's remember that my doctor says I cannot work, my immunologist says I cannot work but Centrelink still thinks I can. Yeah, I still can't wrap my head around that one. The lady who looks after me at the employment agency is lovely and sees I am struggling. I'm guessing the crying at times gives it away. I was asked if I would like to see a counsellor; I thought, yes please, at least that will give the family a break from all of my yakking and may even help me to mentally and emotionally stay above it all. Thinking that a counsellor was different to a psychiatrist and a psychologist, I walked in for my first session and told the woman I had no interest in seeing a psychiatrist or a psychologist. The young woman replied, "I am a psychologist". Yeah, that was a wee bit awkward. I then chatted to her about *that* psychiatrist I had dealt with in the past. You know this woman was lovely. It was nice to chat to someone other than family. It was good to get some stuff out that I don't want to burden family or friends with. I have had some great fears throughout this journey, so it was good to talk it out. I have been very blessed to have love around me always, my tribe always listens to my yakking, but some thoughts I don't want to worry them with.

February ended with us getting through all the money and car issues and I am still off BHRT and feeling ok. And no more communication from the superannuation company. As for Ms Menopause, well she is just slothing on the lounge. Actually she is not looking as strong as she used to. Interestingly though, I have noticed that she hasn't as many troops around her now. Insomnia, Depression, Electric Shocks, Excessive Fatigue, Feelings of Dread, Inability to Cope, Increase in Allergies and a few more have "left the building." Yeah, I told them all ages ago that I would be packing their bags and kicking them out onto the kerb, I just didn't realise it would be done so quietly. They didn't even put up a fight. Oh don't worry Ms Menopause, I know now that you will be in my life long term, but from what I am seeing it seems we are starting to get a better understanding of each other. That is you in the backseat of my life and me in the driver's seat again. You are not a battle ground for me anymore. I have a new battle to fight and that is with Mr Steroid, or should I just call you by your first name? Prednisone.

March 2015: I have been off my BHRT for a month now and am feeling ok. My skin is holding up and I am not swelling. Hmm, ok maybe I can do without the BHRT a bit longer. Or so I thought but I will get to that a little later. I sent an email to the superannuation company in the first few days of March asking for an update on the status of my claim. It is now two years since I submitted this claim and is it is ten weeks since I saw the immunologist. I received a reply explaining that they were still trying to obtain the report and perhaps I could help them to get it. Yep, true story! Now the superannuation company and the insurance company want me to assist them in getting the report. Unfortunately, further into March my skin started to flare again. It started to swell and the inflammation set in once more. At times my skin was so red and raw I had to lie down with icepacks on my skin to alleviate the pain. Now I am still on steroids, the only thing that I stopped was the BHRT. I stopped the BHRT as I wanted to help out with household bills, but what I didn't realise at the time was that once again I was my own experiment and this again proved that BHRT works. Let's remember that during menopause we lose approximately sixty percent of our oestrogen and all of our progesterone. And remember that progesterone is an anti-inflammatory hormone. Without my natural progesterone, BHRT, my skin was flaring up again. So off I went to my compounder mates at the chemist to get me some more BHRT.

I did end up ringing my immunologist's receptionist. I am over this crap. I had a good chat with her, saying at the end that waiting fourteen weeks for a report to be completed and sent to the insurance company is not acceptable. Fourteen bloody weeks! I have great respect for this immunologist but fourteen weeks, how do they think this is ok? Not long after, I received a message as I had missed the call. It was my immunologist ringing me to chat. At first I thought, gulp, he's gonna want a piece of me, but then I thought I don't care, busy or not busy don't these specialists even consider the families who are waiting on these reports? It's just so feckin beyond me.

So I rang him back. He was really lovely and he apologised for the misunderstanding and said that the report had been sent to the appropriate person at the insurance company on the 2nd of March 2015. The misunderstanding he was talking about was when his receptionist told me it had not been done yet. I also told him that the insurance company is still claiming they have not received it. Ok, so I saw him on the 23rd of December 2014 and the report was sent on the 2nd of March 2015. Still a good ten weeks up the track. I do understand these specialists get busy, but my advice would be don't take on more than you can handle. His receptionist, when giving me the wrong information, whined that he does so many of these reports. What I really want to say to her now is, "So what? I am talking to you about my report."

Next port of call was the superannuation fund. I rang them with the information my immunologist had given me. I got a call back from them the next day saying it had not been received. I think I may have even hissed, "Fix it then!" We are now coming to the end of March. As you are now aware, this is the cycle. I deal with my superannuation company and they deal with the insurance company. Whilst talking to the woman who handles my claim she made a comment regarding the insurance company, it was like she was trying to make them sound good. All I could say was, "The insurance company has never exceeded my expectations!" Really? After all this crap being thrown around again you are trying to give me a pep talk? Tell someone who cares because right now all I care about is getting my claim paid so it can take the pressure off my family financially and emotionally. Neither of you, my Superannuation Company and Insurance Company, has given me anything but stress, which has done nothing, but hinder my recovery and exhaust my loved ones who have cared for me.

April 2015: Now I am back on my BHRT and will never go off it again. I am over the synthetic steroids, I will be glad to see the day when all I need is BHRT. My skin is clearing up, I am not swelling as much nor am I as red. I love you BHRT! I went off it for two months so I've got to expect it to take a bit of time to settle down again. My greatest battle now is getting off the Prednisone and seeing if A1 and A2 can kick in and live all by themselves again.

Now as you know we are all using one car. Yes it came back fixed – well, bandaged as well as possible - until I get more funds to put into it. I had an appointment to go to and was dropping the daughter off at work on the way. We are now in mid-April. As I walked to the car I checked our mailbox. In it was an express post envelope from my superannuation company. You know, I was too scared to open it. I sat there waiting for the daughter, trying to prepare myself for them denying my claim. I just kept fumbling with the envelope, and then I saw on the back it stated it was documents. Hey why would they send me documents if they had denied my claim? As the daughter walked to the car I showed her the envelope and let her open it. The insurance company had finally, after two years and two months, finally paid my claim. I was so happy! It doesn't fix my health but what it does do is take away the worry of money and, most importantly, it eases the financial burden on my beautiful family. Wow, the day finally came. I still do not understand how an insurance company is allowed to take so long to pay a claim. Perhaps that is something I will look into when I feel better.

So documents and all the other things that are required are sent back with a request that a copy of the immunologist's report is sent to my family doctor. There was still a bit of mucking around for a good week, someone went on leave, blah, so I'm not going to believe it until I have that money in my bank account.

May 2015: Unfortunately right at the beginning of May we were flooded and had to be evacuated. Our home is highset and some in the street wanted to stay, but when you have an SES guy in a canoe paddling past your home and his opinion is to go… well we went! We were also allowed to take our cat. "Cat?" I hear you all say. Yes our beautiful cat, but you get to know her better shortly. I wasn't leaving without her. So once she was comfy in her cat cage, we all had a trip in a canoe to dry land. We sat in an ambulance as it was a bit cold. We were then taken to emergency accommodation in a police car and the motel we stayed in for the night allowed us to bring the cat. I was just thankful that she didn't make a mess anywhere. It was a bit strange walking out to the front desk in the morning carrying the cat amongst all these people in suits etc, but hey…. We had to get home and we always get a bit of a giggle out of the silliness of things at times.

Fortunately, it didn't affect the top part of our home but I am 5ft 2 in and I would have drowned in that water, that's how far it came up. I know here in Australia we now talk in metres, but I am still 5ft 2in tall.

When we did get home we were advised that some other animals in the street didn't make it which was sad, but otherwise we are all ok. It's just a matter of catching our breath and cleaning up. And for the first and only time I will state that I am glad there was a bit of mucking around on the superannuation company's part because if they had sent the cheque when it should have been, it may have gone down with the flood as the flood water was also in our letter box.

So there was one more call from the woman handling my case telling me the cheque should have been sent by now, and the next day, after her doing some chasing up, we received it in the mail. So we went from being traumatised by the flood to being ecstatic that the battle for my claim had finally ended. Before the conversation ended with the superannuation woman she said, "This is a good outcome for you." All I could say was "No. This is the right outcome for me." So it has now taken two years and three months for my claim to be paid. I understand these companies have to be sure they're not just giving money away willy-nilly, but same old same old, I still do not understand how they are allowed to take so long to pay out a claim.

I am very grateful that battle is over, but I realise that these funds are not going to last forever, so I still say to the tribe, "Now we all start seriously saving again!" I have now been battling this ill health for nearly five years and I haven't been able to work for two years and ten months. The slog to get my mojo back is not over, I know that, but taking the worry of money out of the equation has to be good for my health I reckon. I have never been materialistic and I have never cared about wealth. Money to me has always meant freedom. Now I have the freedom to just concentrate on my health for a little while. I have the freedom to pay back debts and get up to date financially. The freedom of being able to pay back what is owed to my tribe is the most joyous thing. My beautiful family now has the freedom to breathe and know all is going to be ok. Yep, the freedom money brings is priceless.

Oh yes and I said a very happy and joyous "see yar, don't want to be yar" to Centrelink! A bit ironic as I think I was on the verge of getting that bloody Disability pension. I am thankful that Centrelink is there in times of need, but the way they treat menopausal women has to change. Actually I think they owe me two days but hey, as soon as I could I ran - well walked - as fast as I could away from them. This also meant that my appointments with the disability employment agency stopped, so to all of you I thank you so much for your support. You knew I was struggling and you were always very compassionate, considerate and kind. Hey, perhaps you could teach Centrelink staff your people skills!

I also had my eyes checked. Prednisone can cause a lot of health problems for your body including your eyes. I had the normal check but also got another test done which looks deeper into your eyes. It was all very interesting. I felt sorry for the young girl doing the test because when she said I need reading glasses but otherwise my eyes are fine, I was so excited that I jumped out of the seat and did a little jig! So I sit here now, proudly wearing my new reading glasses in the knowledge that this is a normal part of being middle aged and not due to damage done by steroids. Suck on that Prednisone!

I need to mention that when I gave the lawyer the flick mid 2014, (not you my first lawyer who I have known for over twenty years, I am talking about the third lawyer,) I sent off a list of questions to the insurance company asking them to "please explain". I asked them why they had not been acting in good faith regarding my claim. I asked them why they were discriminating against me as a menopausal woman. Yep, because that is exactly how I was being treated. Anyhoo that battle, thank god, is done and dusted. I seriously wonder if we may be seeing a hell of a lot more of these claims if women are not educated more about menopause. What the heck, perhaps there may even be some court cases over the way they are treated throughout their menopause. I dunno, just sayin'.

The end of May saw me finally organising the editing of my book.

June 2015: Winter has started here in Australia. I get a little worried as last year my 'flu and cold started in June and didn't end until September with an admission to hospital in between, so I am really hoping and praying that doesn't all repeat itself this winter, only time will tell.

So June brings no more dealings with the insurance company, someone with the expertise is now tidying up my book for publication, and our much loved "renovators dream home" has started to get some work done on it. My brother and daughter forfeited having cars just to help keep this little tribe together, but now they have a car and my car went back in for some serious work. Some have said that the money I spend on getting my car fixed will cost more than the car is worth but I don't care. My car is staying. As I mentioned, it used to be my sister's car before we lost her to leukaemia, and I always feel closer to her when I am in it. I know to some these cars may sound materialistic, but to me they are a necessity and well deserved. We all pulled together throughout the toughest part of this journey and we made it! Well the whole feckin journey was tough. I love you my little tribe and what I am able to give back to you now has delighted me.

I know I still have more ahead of me health-wise, but how humbling and wonderful is it to know that my little family stayed by my side all the way through this. I know for a fact that I would never have made it this far without their love and care. They always kept me safe as much as possible, and as much as we had to tighten our belts and go without, not once did they ever complain. I have to say though there is a lot of stuff one can go without and there are many different dishes that can be made with mince meat. My personal favourite? Rissoles!

So here I am in June 2015 and still on 4.5mg of steroids. Yes, since being advised by the immunologist in December 2014 to go back up to 5mg as usual, it has been an up and down journey with Prednisone. I know at one time I planned to be off them in September. Actually I planned that a few times, but they are really hard to get off once you have been on them long term. It can be quite dangerous if I come off them too fast. So this plan is to hopefully be off them by Christmas Eve, but again it will be a waiting game.

June also saw me heading in to my family doctor with a big basket of fruit and some cup cakes to say thank you to him for all his care, advice and respect. It was also for the nurses who gave my injections as well as some cupcakes for the front desk girls. We went through a bit of the immunologist's report but it was huge! My doctor said the full report was nearly a book. Ha! What was interesting is that through all the crap with the insurance company, it was always about me never being able to work again for the claim to be paid. I always felt this was a little unrealistic. I had even said to my immunologist that it seemed to be a big ask of him to state, "Jenni will NEVER work again." How would he know that? Actually the only one who would know that is the man upstairs. Yes, I am ill and it may be a long-term thing, but what a situation for the insurance company to put the immunologist in.

Anyhoo getting back to the report. It was too big to go through it all but it mentioned that my adrenal glands may take another one or two years to function by themselves again. I wasn't too happy when we read that, but it also stated that perhaps in the future I may be able to return to work in a smaller capacity. So, after all those years of mucking around with the insurance company and them trying not to pay my claim, they now have paid it out even though a specialist's opinion is that I may be able to return to work in the future. Don't get me wrong, I am glad to hear this but geez almighty, why then all the unnecessary stress and crap we have had to deal with for all those years with that lot?

I also had a bit of an interesting chat to the nurses. When I was finished seeing my doctor I needed to go to the ladies, and on the way through three nurses were gathered. Two were my injection nurses and one a training nurse. On seeing me, one of the nurses came up and gave me a hug and thanked me for the fruit and cakes. This nurse then hung her arm over my shoulder and started telling the trainee nurse that a few years ago after a flood, when they thought my vials of cocktail for my desensitization injections may have been spoiled due to having no electricity for a while, I was the only one who didn't complain. This nurse said I took it all in my stride. What a nice story. Apparently the other patients who kept their cocktail vials at this medical centre gave them all a hard time. Oh well, I was probably just exhausted from whinging about so much other stuff in my writings!

I also got the results of a chest x-ray, blood tests, pap-smear test and abdominal ultrasound. All have come back ok. I also had a two yearly mammogram and am waiting on those results. It took three attempts by three nurses to take my blood for these tests. The first just couldn't get a vein. The second blew my vein up in my hand. That was really interesting though, I never knew veins were so tough and could blow up like that! My vein had to be ice packed and bandaged and I was a wee bit bruised from it. I felt a bit sorry for the nurses as they felt pretty bad, but I just reassured them that they had done their best and that was all I could ask. It did worry me a bit though when it was suggested that I might have to have blood taken from between my toes! Yeahnah, that ain't happening. So after a bit of a break I went back to the usual place where my blood is drawn. The third was the nurse who usually takes my blood but she had been away. Her first attempt was successful. It got to the stage that I wanted to scream, "SOMEONE TAKE MY BLOOD WILL YAR!" When I reached home I let my facebook mates, yes all ten of them, know that all was good with the results. One of the comments received from a lovely mate made me sit back and think though. This beautiful friend simply said, "Does that mean I can come and visit now?"

Yeah, it really tore at my heartstrings. I have been so zoned in on just working so hard on my health and to just continue to "be" that I really didn't think that anyone would be missing me. I have had friends try to keep in contact but I just wasn't well enough. I have had a friend just walk away, which I do understand, as some just cannot deal with the massiveness of illness at times. Plus I never wanted anyone's life to be put on hold just because I am sick. I have always been a self-contained little unit. Oh okay, maybe a little needy at times in my younger years, but I didn't realise, except for the fabulous tribe, how much of a lone wolf I had become. So I say to my beautiful mate, "I never meant to lose sight of any of you. Just existing and continuing to 'be' became my full time job. Hopefully though I will see you all at the fifty-five and still alive party." Yeah, hopefully that party will be a sure thing now!

Just getting back to that chat I had with the nurses, when she was telling that story where I said "My first allergist", emphasizing the first. We then got into a chat about Ms Menopause - of course! It is just interesting to see women's reactions to menopause at times. One of the older nurses said after a bit, "I don't feel comfortable talking about Menopause," but then went straight on to talk about men's prostate problems. So I did my usual spiel that went like this: "I get that some men may have prostate problems, but the only sure thing in the human race is that every woman will go through menopause, and it needs to stop being a taboo subject and be put out there in the wider community so women will feel more comfortable talking about it." We all continued to chat for a bit more then with another hug off I went. Yeah it surprises me. Don't get me wrong, I believe every woman has the right to go through menopause exactly as she chooses, whether it is quietly, loudly or whatever. What I don't want is women not talking about menopause and suffering in silence because that is the way it has always been, and they have been made to feel uncomfortable speaking about it. I also found it interesting that she was quite comfortable talking about a man's prostate but not comfortable talking about menopause. It seemed to me that once again menopause was downplayed and I noted how easily the chat had changed to men's prostates. I don't want my menopause compared to "maybe a man may have prostate problems", and I sure as hell don't ever again want my menopause compared to a sprained ankle! Yeah true story, but out of great respect for that person, that is as much as I say in regard to the "ankle" comparison.

I also saw my BHRT doctor again. So exciting! I hadn't seen him for a while due to lack of funds, but fortunately I was able to get my BHRT and natural steroid scripts from my family doctor. I just wanted to touch base with him and see if we can come up with a plan to finally get me out of the grip of Prednisone. I had a chat with him about the time last year when my estrogen level went up naturally by itself. I don't know if I mentioned this. I had actually been thinking that maybe I had produced estrogen naturally due to using the natural progesterone. To recap a bit; when the adrenal glands need to produce more estrogen they call on progesterone and steal from it, as they don't give back to progesterone. Just as I was getting a bit excited about my theory, my BHRT doctor explained that the more body fat we have, the more estrogen our body produces. Hmm ok, then all I could do was pat my gut. At least that explained that. I am now going down 0.5mg every three to four weeks and my BHRT doctor has given me another herb to add to the natural steroids I am on which I start when I get to 4mgs. I am really hoping this works. The only synthetic thing I am on now is Prednisone and I can't wait to kick him to the kerb too. Why is Prednisone a "him"? Well Prednisone sounds like a Spanish man to me.

We also discussed my tooth, yeah still walking around with my front tooth missing. I explained to him what had been said to me about the adrenal crisis etc. He wasn't totally convinced, so we are now waiting for him to get a copy of the immunologist's report and I will head back in the next couple of months and hopefully get that sorted.

Unfortunately, a little while after seeing my doctors I started to get a bit sniffly. Yeah this is what I was hoping would not happen. Look I am ok if I get a 'flu in winter like the majority of Aussies, a 'flu that comes and goes and doesn't linger for three months. But I guess I just have to wait and see where it goes.

Actually it didn't take long to see where it went. I was watching a movie a few nights later and all of a sudden my head just felt like it was whirling. I was ok, but it felt strange, then I started getting a headache. I woke the next morning feeling off but it was the day after that it hit me. I woke up with a congested chest which, when I coughed, felt like it was being hit by a hammer. I had a nose full of snot, my sinuses were hurting and swollen, and my voice sounded like a mixture of that of a deep husky transvestite and a fourteen year old boy whose voice was getting ready to break, that is if my voice was even there! Where the hell did that come from? Was it from sitting in two doctors' waiting rooms? Was it the hug I received from one of the daughter's friends who had the sniffles? One never says no to a hug regardless of how down and out one's immune system is, unless I am in hospital and that no-no has been issued by a doctor. Or is this due to going down 0.5mg of Prednisone steroid? Who feckin knows?

Fortunately, I was able to get in and see my family doctor. After the usual checks and questions I was put on a course of antibiotics. The funny thing is though, as I write this a few days later I am not suffering as much as I thought I would. My chest is ok now, well not as sore, still a bit snotty in the nose, I'm sleeping a bit more but otherwise I am ok. But I have learnt not to get too excited. Even my family doctor said I was still brighter than last year and he reminded me of how I was at that time… shiver! The only thing my doctor said that I didn't like was, "You will have to go up on your steroids to help you get through this."

Well out came the folded arms, I slumped into the chair and suddenly turned into a thirteen-year-old teenage girl with attitude. I had the screwed up nose, the only thing I was missing was the chewing gum. I think I had another reaction last year to this comment too! In my head I was thinking, "Nah don't wanna!"

Once I put my attitude away we discussed it. He is right, he is just ensuring that I am ok but I am not happy about it. I have been on these things for four years next month, all because I am menopausal, unbelievable. So I did increase my steroids but not the Prednisone ones. I went up on my natural steroids, the Adrenotone ones. I have been taking four of these daily and started on six daily when I got home. I know I am safe to do this as when I was first put on them by my BHRT doctor ages ago I started on six. I can live with that but I'm not telling my doctor. I do respect his professional opinion but I need to get out of the grip of Prednisone. If I splatter well I have only one person to blame and that is me, but at the same time I've got to be given the chance to see if I can get off them.

So to end June 2015 I am still dealing with this 'flu a bit better but still chesty, snotty and feeling like crap. Interestedly though, I met up with a woman I used to work with many years ago and we had a bit of a chinwag. This woman and her partner also have the 'flu and she is just coming out of it after two weeks, so as much I am sorry that she too has suffered through the 'flu, it actually gave me hope that maybe I might be just like the everyday Aussie who gets a it. Again only time will tell. I also received my breast screening results back and all is good. Thanks God, appreciate it!

I hadn't been dealing with swelling for a while but on the last day of June I woke up swollen. I was quite despondent about this as I just couldn't work out what had triggered it. I need to know I am getting better and when this happens, granted it is only on the odd day now, it tends to pull me down emotionally and mentally. Of course it all has to do with my immune system and my adrenal glands but I don't want this to happen! I need to know that I have lived my eighties in my fifties and that I can look forward to living my fifties in my eighties - well you know what I mean. I guess the only positive is that for whatever reason, this is the first time I have swollen up in quite a while. I also had to stop the antibiotics that my doctor gave me, as a few days after starting them I felt nauseated.

The end of June also saw me buying a second hand treadmill. Yeah, the walking was becoming non-existent again and I know how important it is to exercise for my health, but when one has adrenal fatigue, and depending on what stage you are at with it, exercise can stress A1 and A2 and can be detrimental to ones health so I will start off slowly and see how it goes. I will say though it is wonderful to just get out of bed, eat to take my medication, then walk down stairs, turn the radio on and hop on the treadmill. I am aware that I need to get sunlight as well for my Vitamin D hit but yeah, this is my type of exercising for now. Maybe one day I will build back up to climbing those mountains of streets that I have in the past.

July 2015: This month actually was quite an emotional roller coaster. Lots to talk about but first I had to say goodbye to one of my facebook mates who lost his battle with cancer. You know I only re-connected with this wonderful soul again in December of last year but by then he had had cancer for a few years. We had dated many, many moons ago before he picked up and moved to America to make his mark on the music industry. I last saw him when he was a young man, then we fast-forwarded and both of us were suddenly middle-aged. I don't know if I have the right, but this is how I felt when I heard he had passed over, DAMN BLOODY ANGRY! Of course I am terribly sad but I just felt so angry that he lost the fight. Not angry with him, just angry that this wonderful soul who was only fifty-five was lost to cancer. I have lost loved ones that I have grieved for and still carry in my heart today but why am I so angry over the loss of this friend? It took a bit of time to subside, actually I can feel it welling up again as I write, but I guess I just wanted him to be a success story. For him, his wife, his family and for me! When I spoke of this to my daughter, who had noticed the effect his loss was having on me, I told her that I know illness does not pick and choose, but it is so unfair and I just wanted him to be a success story. I needed to hear a story of success against illness! My daughter responded with, "You will be your own success story against illness." This comment was taken in and held close to my heart. I am filled with so much love and admiration for this young woman. Thank you daughter, you will never really know how much that one sentence meant to me. I still feel the anger and even anxiety of losing this amazing man to cancer but am so thankful that he had his beautiful wife and sister by his bedside. See you on the other side my facebook friend. Don't get too excited though I ain't planning to meet up with you again for a good thirty-odd Earth years, but I will now carry you in my heart too and I will always remember you as being the first to take me to see Billy Joel in concert all those many years ago.

I also had my first night out since Ms Menopause knocked back in 2010. The daughter, seeing I was upset about my friend, took me to see a Divinyls Tribute show. I was a bit nervous and still sitting with the 'flu. Yeah, another dose of it when the tribe brought it home. The hair has been dyed again without any reaction, and I decided I felt I was well enough to give it a go and head out to the Divinyls Tribute. And so I did. I sat through it all and enjoyed it; I was well enough to be there! And this made me think. I know I have spoken of getting there but not really knowing where there is, well after this night out I found where there is. "There" is my life, and getting back into the world. It was lovely to be back out *there*. I know I am still not well enough to be who I used to be, but just getting a very small feel of it again felt wonderful. Oh and I guess when I do get there again I have to remember I am now five years older. Oh well, who cares! Actually I am deliriously happy that I will be five years older since the beginning of this whole journey with Ms Menopause. I am thankful to still be here to be able to get there, I am able to still "be," so roll on the next chapters of my life, here's to living the rest of my life healthily, happily and disgracefully.

Even though I am dealing with the 'flu I have noticed other differences this winter compared to last year, besides my weird sense of humour returning. I am staying awake for a full day, I have more energy, and my walking on the treadmill continues without any more inflammation. I don't feel as ill on a daily basis even though I am still struggling with the 'flu due to my immune system. I feel and know that I am still not "me" again health wise, and I know I am not at the stage where I can hit the ground running yet, but I am definitely doing better, so far, than last year. I can't wait to feel like me again. I can't wait to feel life again instead of just doing life. I can't wait until my soul fully awakens and I can head towards my old age capable and happy. I know I perhaps should not get too excited yet but, I yam what I yam and I yam excited to think and feel that maybe my life is waiting for me in the not too distant future. E X C I T I N G!

I had been waiting for the movie *Still Alice* to come out on DVD. I haven't gone to see a movie with a crowd for ages. The way my immune system has been it would only take someone coughing out of the window of their car without covering their mouth as they drove past the movie theatre for me to get sick, so yeah, not happening yet! I was hoping this movie would confirm a few things that I have spoken about, and it did. Without giving anything away, this story is based on a woman who heads into Alzheimer's, oh, oops sorry, just gave it away. I understand that in this movie her diagnosis is genetic but I found it very interesting that when she knew something was wrong she visited her specialist and one of the first questions he asked her was, "Are you menopausal?" Hmmm interesting.

The second confirmation came when she visited a home for Alzheimer's patients and it was mentioned that the majority of residents were women. So this confirms for me that the medical world does know that menopause can lead to Alzheimer's disease but they still try and ignore it! This isn't me just yakking about it Medical Community, this is in a movie being watched by millions of people. This movie was very raw and sad and scary and very close to the bone as we see how a menopausal woman uneducated about menopause may be affected by it.

Chapter 48

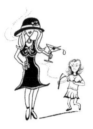

THE HORMONES OF A TWENTY-ONE-YEAR-OLD

"Huh?" I hear you say. What has this to do with Menopause? Well get yourself comfy and I will tell you. You know I just felt a twinge of sadness, as this will be the last time I ask you to get comfy.

This young woman has been a friend, ex-friend and friend of my daughter's for a good few years. When I first met her she was a funny, sociable young woman, well that's what I saw as a parent. As time went on she was in and out of our lives, but when she would stay with us I started to notice that her moods were quite erratic and this was affecting her relationships, and she even seemed depressed at times. This young one also dropped quite a bit of weight. Now I know that many of you may be thinking, "So? She lost weight." Granted, but I could see and feel that this wasn't healthy weight loss. I told my daughter I was concerned about her and asked both the girls to have pap smear tests, yeah and that was like asking them to cut their own arm off and chew on it slowly! They did have their pap smears though and both came back ok, thank God, because cancer was starting to swirl around in my head concerning the twenty-one year old. Not my daughter, she is the twenty-three year old. Ok, so I got that wrong I thought, and was very happy I was wrong. But the twenty-one year old still isn't well from what I am observing so I then started asking her a few questions.

She told me that she was having trouble sleeping, and that she would get really hot in bed and start sweating to the extent where she would have to kick her covers off even if it was cold weather. Her energy levels were pretty well non-existent to the point where she was finding it hard to get out of bed, and her periods were erratic. I am watching this go down and I am thinking, "You sound like you are menopausal."

Now I know I am all about menopause, and yes I am sure I even get annoying at times, but to me, she was showing signs of hormonal imbalance. I asked her if I could take her to my family doctor to get some tests done and off we went. Now before I continue, this young woman had been bounced from pillar to post when it came to seeing doctors. She knew something was wrong but all the doctors and the specialist she had seen were never able to tell her what was going on. Yes, they were quick to try and stick her on anti-depressants and even label her bipolar.

So now we are at my family doctor's and I asked him if he could please do a blood test to check this young woman's hormones. He was a bit hesitant due to the "only twenty-one" fact, and he said that it would not be her hormones. Well I guess you all know me by now, so I shot back to him, "How do you know it's not her hormones until you do a blood test?" Blood tests were done and yep, one of her hormones was out of whack, or we were told it was one hormone at the time.

Moving on. I always knew that when I had the funds I would be taking her to see my BHRT doctor, so off we went. When he saw her hormone results he was shocked. This young woman's oestrogen was out of kilter, her progesterone was pretty well non-existent and another hormone was showing an abnormal amount as well. This poor sweetheart had been suffering all this time because not one feckin' doctor would take the time to look into her ills thoroughly. My BHRT doctor was a bit annoyed that not one other doctor had helped this twenty-one-year-old. All I could say was, "I don't think any doctors know much about a woman's hormones." My BHRT replied, "They are given the basics." I then asked my BHRT doctor whether this could send this twenty-one year old into early menopause. He felt that it wouldn't even though she had started to show signs of menopause, but if it had not been looked into now it could have turned into cancer. Yep, said right in front of the twenty-one year old and the middle-aged woman. I don't know who was more shocked, the twenty-one year old or the fifty-four year old. So the cancer concerns for this young woman were real.

Of course my BHRT doctor got straight on to it. First a more up to date blood test, then once that was received he put her on some natural tablets to help get her periods back to a normal monthly cycle, and she is now also on BHRT.

Do you know how she got into this mess that could have turned into cancer? When she was twelve she had her first period. Apparently her periods were a bit hit and miss at times and they could be quite constant periods when she first reached puberty. The doctor she was taken to back then, instead of perhaps waiting to see if her body was just trying to find it's natural cycle, put the twelve-year-old, I repeat *the twelve-year-old*, on the pill. Not an oral pill but the one that is inserted into the skin for three feckin' years! Then when this was removed she was given another hormone injection. Unbelievable! So from twelve to fifteen, the inserted hormone, then a whack of more hormone crap by injection. No wonder she is having hormone problems now. *Doctors have to be made more accountable for the way they treat women, from puberty to menopause.*

It upsets me so much to think that this once happy young woman could have been dealing with cancer thanks to the incompetence of the medical world. Words cannot describe the fear I feel if we didn't get on top of it now. Wow I need to shake that off quick smart. Just writing about it makes my blood boil.

The twenty-one-year-old is relieved to know that it's not just all in her head as suggested by some of the doctors. Hey Doc, FECK OFF! She has finally found a doctor who sees it for what it is: her hormones! I can't help thinking about my BHRT doctor saying, "They are given the basics." Why are doctors only given basic information on women's hormones? It's ludicrous. So many women are suffering as a result of the medical community's incompetence, yeah things are going to change and while I have breath left in me it is going to happen in my lifetime. I need to get stronger in mind, body and soul, physically, emotionally and mentally, so that when I come up against the medical world I will ensure I will be able to hold my own. Yeah, the way I am working my treadmill I may even be able to out run them if needed!

My BHRT doctor also told us a really interesting fact. When I first started BHRT he told me I couldn't overdose my body on it so I told this to the twenty-one-year-old, but this time my BHRT doctor said, "Yes you can." Huh? Of course I questioned him on this conflicting information. It turns out that one can overdose on it but it would have to be really high amounts. He went on to say that when women are pregnant, their progesterone goes up about 200 times the normal amount, and their immune system is suppressed so the baby does not get rejected. I have mentioned this earlier. Wow, the body is such an amazing thing. It makes sense that progesterone would increase at this time of a woman's life. Why? Well, when the immune system is suppressed in pregnancy it becomes easier to catch colds and illnesses, and inflammation in other parts of the body will occur. With the progesterone increasing in pregnancy, that balances what is needed in the body while the immune system is suppressed... clear as mud? Actually I remember a while ago that the medical profession was giving progesterone to some pregnant woman to help stop miscarriages.

I remember this as I thought at the time, "Interesting but I bet the progesterone they are using is the synthetic one and not the natural BHRT progesterone I am on." So to recap, the only overdose or side effects of BHRT are headaches or sore boobs. There is that saliva test you can do to see how much progesterone you have in your body and also a blood test will give you a reading. Even at the time I had too much progesterone in my body I did suffer severe headaches, but once you tweak it, nothing will slow you down!

So to end July, which has felt like a few months crammed into one, it has now been three years since I had to walk from my job. I am down to 3.5mg of Prednisone and am holding ok. I feel like I am coming out of the 'flu, yahoo, one month earlier than last year, but as usual we will wait and see. Am I in my healing stage? I am not fully back until I am off steroids but some days I feel that I need to be doing more, well not need, but feel like I want to do more. I am getting out into the world a bit more and have even bumped into people I knew before all of this crap. The main question I'm asked is, "Are you back at work?" I haven't the will to tell them that I actually never stopped working, it was just that this "job" was the fight for my life. So I just say, "No, but I have written a book that is coming out next year." That is enough to shock them and divert the conversation! Ha!

I used to feel weird saying, "I wrote a book." Who Me? Naah! But yes, and why not? Now I say it with confidence. I believe in this book, it is my truth, so yeah I need to give it the respect it deserves. I wrote a book and I am very proud of it. There is no sex in it, no snogging Who, who now, who is always right, or who always wanted sex when all I wanted was a hug. No travelling the world to find one's self, as Ms menopause put a pause to all of that fun. It is simply one woman's journey with Ms Menopause and who is going to get the truth out there!

August 2015: Roll on August! Yes! I was just going to count the days down, all seemed to be fine. Yahoo I thought! My final month of writing. I'm going to get through August without any incidents, right? Well, no! My teeth started to ache. Yep, why not? Everything else was looking pretty damn positive! My face started to swell, not the cute "Who from Whoville look", just a swollen face and I was in so much pain! I know that I am supposed to be careful with extractions due to my adrenal fatigue, but I really was put between a rock and a hard place. I did get antibiotics from my doctor who explained to me that if I didn't get my teeth looked at now it could cause other complications such as blood poisoning or even cause problems with my jaw bone - feckin fabulous!

I drove away from that appointment knowing I had made the decision to get some extractions done. I don't do toothache well, I can deal with a lot but toothache nearly brings me to my knees. I also knew that after making the appointment with the dentist and whilst driving there, A1 and A2 were shivering in their little adrenal skins with their little white knuckles clenched with fear! "Sorry guys I know we have worked so hard to get you both healthy and active again, but I haven't got a choice on this one. And no! Blood poisoning or my jaw dropping out of my face is not an option! Geez I nurture you two back to the best health that I can and yet you can so easily visualize me without a feckin jaw? Look I know you two are scared, so am I, but right now I haven't got a choice."

The dentist was great. After I explained to him all about my adrenal glands we went ahead and had six injections and four teeth pulled. Yep! I personally am happy to start this, but I am concerned about A1 and A2. I now understand why I had to wait. My immunologist had told me that I would need to go up on my steroids if I had extractions or I would have to wait, but he never explained why. I also never thought to ask. Well I now know. The dentist explained that the needles I had to have make your heart pump faster which in turn gives you an adrenalin rush. No wonder for the next few weeks my lower back was aching and I felt a bit groggy, as no doubt I had just given A1 and A2 a near death experience! Geez almighty. They are supposed to be healing and stressing less, then along comes this almighty adrenalin rush. I am so, so sorry guys, just keep hanging in there. Oh and did you see anything on the other side A1 or A2? Ok, no, it's not funny, I get it. A friend asked if I had the happy gas, well firstly it wasn't offered, the dentist went straight in with the six needles, and personally I don't like having gas at the dentist, I am too scared that I might give away too much whilst under the influence.

So I am dealing with this then the daughter comes home not feeling well. A tribe member takes her to our doctor as her asthma is playing up. Our doctor then gets her whisked away to hospital by ambulance, yep another "it doesn't rain, but it pours" moment in our family. Our daily paper is screaming out on the front page, *BRISBANE FLU FIASCO, WORST OUTBREAK IN YEARS*. It is a different strain of 'flu this year, which is hitting people a lot harder. Of course it is! I just feckin wanted to count down the days of August gently and quietly, eh Guv, but nah! Oh, how selfish of me, back to the daughter. Thank God her partner had the day off and was able to meet the daughter at the hospital. You know a relationship is special when one is wiping spew from their partner's mouth eh?

The medical team at the hospital tried to tell my daughter she was dealing with anxiety! Yep, true story. Idiots! And a bloody dangerous diagnosis. Look I get that when my daughter is struggling to breathe due to her asthma, that an emotional anxiety could be in play as well, who wouldn't get a wee bit anxious NOT BEING ABLE TO BREATHE! Anyhoo, my daughter, knowing that her asthma has been triggered by something else, tells the doctor that she needs antibiotics. I also understand the whole "if it's a viral infection, antibiotics won't help", but as explained to the doctor by the daughter, she was also coughing up yucky stuff. The end result was that my daughter was well enough to come home without being admitted. She had antibiotics in hand but it was taking a while for her to pick up so off she went back to our doctor who had to give her more antibiotics. As she walked back in the front door after that consultation she also brought "Wheezy Bronchitis" with her. Yep, that too is doing the rounds with the whole Brisbane 'flu fiasco. It took weeks for my daughter to recover from this and did I get it as well? Of course! It was terrible. It made me think that my comment back in July where I said I was coming out of the 'flu one month earlier this year was a crock of crap.

Before going on I just want to tell you a true story in relation to the daughter's admittance to hospital in August last year. The whole "anxiety" diagnosis reminded me of it. When the daughter was admitted last year and before I went up to visit her - you remember, that was when all the germs lurking in the hospital jumped me all at the same time - we spoke on the phone and she told me that the nurses were doing finger pricks on a regular basis to check her blood. Hmm, ok I thought, at least they are being thorough I guess, but I was a little confused about the need for this. When I visited my daughter the tea lady arrived and put a packet of biscuits on the tray. I don't know what made me see it but I noticed they were biscuits that are normally given to people who are diabetic. This is how the rest of it went:

Me: Why are you giving my daughter diabetic biscuits?

Tea Lady: Because she is diabetic.

Me: No she isn't. [The nurse was also in the room] My daughter is not diabetic.

Nurse: Oh we were just keeping an eye on her sugar levels to see if we need to give her insulin. [Nurse turns to daughter] You are not diabetic?

Me: You will not be giving her any insulin until we speak to the doctor. The daughter has never been and is not now a DIABETIC!

Bloody unbelievable! The Nurse then walked out of the room mumbling that she will look into it. Of course I followed her out and asked her if she realised how dangerous it could have been if they had given my daughter insulin because they thought she was diabetic! I also told her that I wanted answers as to why my daughter was even given this diagnosis. We never got a straight answer about this mix up, all that was said was that the woman at reception had thought she'd overheard that the daughter was diabetic. What a crock of crap! Unbelievable! You know what I reckon happened? Pure incompetence on their part and bloody dangerous too. The more dealings I have with the medical community at times, the more scared I get thinking that these are the people we trust with our lives when we are sick and highly vulnerable. I was going to make a complaint but I just wanted to get the daughter home safely and then I splattered under the strain of having all those hospital germs sitting on me like a monkey on my back.

Now to do a quantum leap forward into now, August 2015. We got through the worst of this years 'flu etc and my teeth healed nicely thank God, but I still get quite despondent when this crap happens. I was chatting to the daughter and I said that "really the teeth stuff could happen to anyone and the flu has happened to many..." Before I could finish my sentence my daughter stated, "Well that makes you normal." The only thing I could think of saying was, "Define normal!" But it's true, I know I have been hit harder due to this journey, but there are so many more positives this year compared to last August.

As sick as I have been, this is the first year since 2011 that I haven't had to go within cooee of a hospital. As soon as I was able, I got back onto my treadmill and have worked my way up to an hour. An hour! Who would have thought? Not me! I actually went out and bought an exercising outfit too, you know the material that when you put it on it makes a snapping noise and attaches itself to your skin? I believe it is called polyester/elastane. It's really nice. Of course it is colourful with splashes of bright colours that actually go well with my black shoes and bright pink socks, lovely. The first time I put it on, it was, as expected, tight in the boobs, belly and bum area, a very attractive look! You know I was looking at this happening before me and I had a thought. I took my wild hair out its ponytail and tussled it more with my fingers and there in my mirror suddenly appeared Edwina, commonly known as Eddy from *Absolutely Fabulous.* Wow! I had my idol standing before me in my mirror! All I needed now was high shoes, a big brimmed, floppy hat, chunky jewellery and a bottle of "Bolly" with a straw in it to complete this whole look. Brings tears to my eyes, such a wonderful moment. If I didn't know that was me standing there I would have been star struck! Yeah Ms Menopause, suck on that. I will morph into whoever I want to morph into, not who you expect me to be. Actually as fabulous as the "Eddy" moment was Ms Menopause, we all know who the long term morphing will be. Yes ME!

Ok, so yes, I have been pretty well sick since June, as I was last year, but even though I plunged into that last 'flu, I still have moments of feeling better. I also think A1 and A2 are going to be ok. I still have more dental work to do, but I am giving us all time to get over that last fright. My skin, besides flaring a wee bit, which I think now had a lot to do with my teeth, has been really good. It is so nice to wake up in the morning and not be aware of the skin I live in. I am back to my last battle and that is still with Prednisone, but I just survived the worst 'flu we have had here in Brisbane since 2009, so Prednisone, start packing your bags too because I want you out of the house by the end of this year. Yes, you heard me right, you and I are not seeing in 2016 together! Oh, and the twenty-one year old with hormonal problems is getting there. Her skin is clearing, she is sleeping better and her monthly period seems to be getting itself together. Still early days I know, but I pray that she will be able to get on top of her health.

So to end August, yes and this story, I am still here. I am stronger than I have been since Ms Menopause knocked on my door all the way back in 2010. Putting the 'flu and the teeth thing aside I am exercising daily, I am living full days again without having to sleep. Don't get me wrong though, I still have days of all consuming tiredness but not as often. I know I am in that in-between stage of not being so sick but knowing that I am still not quite there. I am not ready to hit the ground running yet but that horrible feeling of exhaustion that has been with me throughout all these years is gone. I am functioning better every day. I have noticed laughter is back in my life and I have started to blare my fabulous eighties music in my car again as yes, at one stage I wasn't even listening to music. I know that BHRT has given me my life back, even saved my life, and prevented other illnesses from rearing their ugly head. A menopausal woman's hormones need to be treated safely and that is the start and finish of it. The best parts are when I see that smile on my daughter's face again that tells me her soul is happy in the knowledge that her strong, happy and funny mum is returning. The other best part of it is that I am a bigger part of my family again and am there for them when I am needed, and you know what? That makes me happy, and until I kick Prednisone out of my home, being there for my family again is the best healthy and happy ending I could have!

Chapter 49

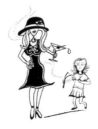

TO BE FOREWARNED IS
TO BE FOREARMED AKA
THE HANDBOOK

I looked into what this actually means and this is what I found:

To know what the enemy is doing is to already have a weapon to use against them. Your insight into their plans gives you an advantage in planning a counter offence and/or defence against an anticipated attack that they don't know you will be aware of.

Basically, you will be going into battle against Ms Menopause. I was attacked by her, I didn't see her coming. I did know she was going to turn up one day, but never would have thought it was going to be such a fight for my life and my whole being. I believe if I already had a weapon to defend myself against her, I would be a lot healthier today. That weapon is knowledge.

I wish this "handbook" had all the answers for you, but I know it hasn't. I hope at least it will give you food for thought and help you in some way as you journey with Ms Menopause. Please, again, be aware that all women will deal with Ms Menopause, but not every woman will have such harsh dealings with her. They say though, that seventy-five to eighty percent of women will have a tough time with her, so better to get prepared, just in case. As I say this, I have searched high and low for that twenty to twenty-five percent of women who have sailed through or have positive stories in relation to menopause, but honestly in all that I have read and with all those I have spoken to so far, I have only found a handful of these women. I do know now that every woman will be affected by her, whether it is at the beginning, during or beyond menopause, when ills blamed on old age really stem from Ms Menopause.

I would also never put women in the same basket. We are all individual and unique. Every woman will deal with this phase of her life in her own way and do what is best for her. Every woman though, will eventually have the same loss of hormones as every other woman on this planet.

It all sounds a bit frightful doesn't it? Years before any symptoms show up our estrogen and progesterone levels are going up and down, a bit like a roller coaster, but remember, the basis of Ms Menopause is that once a woman has her last period, her ovaries produce less estrogen and lose all of their progesterone. We know now of the disastrous and debilitating ripple effect that losing these two hormones has on an otherwise healthy woman, so we need to get these hormones back into our bodies safely, and the earlier you do this the better off you will be. After learning about estrogen dominance, I now know the importance of getting progesterone back into our bodies.Please don't forget for even a moment though that this is your life and your body. If you have insight into how Ms Menopause really can attack you, you will have the advantage of preparing for her knock on the door years before she turns up. This in itself will take away a large slice of the unnecessary suffering.

Also remember, you have a right to question your doctor or anyone about your treatment; you know what you are going through. Demand to be listened to. Hold your head up high whilst you are dealing with Ms Menopause, it's nothing to be ashamed of. I must admit that in the early stages of my acquaintance with her, I used to say I was going through menopause without any feeling or conviction. Now I say it loud and proud, hell yeah! I have earned this right to go through it, but I also have earned the right to go through it in a state of health.

I am very thankful and very blessed that I have been given the opportunity to make it into my fifties and hopefully more. It is meant to be a celebration of our lives, a time where we no longer have to deal with periods, birth control or teenagers, oh, did I say that out aloud? Yahoo!

After finding out that it is the hormones estrogen and progesterone and a bit of testosterone we lose during menopause, I now know there are three stages to Ms Menopause. They are:

1. Perimenopause: Remember how I said that Ms Menopause can be hanging around for years before you even know? Well this is that time. It is when the ovarian hormone levels start changing. Oestrogen and progesterone levels start to decline, but do so unevenly. This is the roller coaster time when our hormones are going up and down. Some symptoms that you may feel or see in this stage are: irregular periods, hot flushes, skin problems, sleep disturbance, mood swings, vaginal dryness and existing conditions and illness rearing up even if they have laid dormant for many years.

   If I had the knowledge I have now back in 2010 I would be a lot healthier today. I was having irregular periods, sleep disturbance, rashes and the "girly bit" could have been suffering with dryness, but I didn't notice. Oh I would have noticed if I was having sex? Oh ok. Who hasn't had a strange period now and then, who hasn't had a sleepless night at times due to thinking too much? As for my rash, I knew I was going to get to it, but I didn't know this was Ms Menopause starting to get to me.

If I had known what I know now, and if everything was going okay up to say, my mid forties, I would have known these were the first signs that Ms Menopause had arrived. If you are being told that Ms Menopause is only about hot flushes and mood swings, just laugh and definitely don't let a doctor turn you away, because he/she thinks you are too young for menopause. I read of a woman who started dealing with Ms Menopause at thirty-two years old. Her doctor was constantly telling her that she was simply too young and sent her on her way. This intelligent woman who knows her own body insisted tests be done. The test came back, of course, showing this young thirty-two year old was menopausal. Again, stand your ground, nobody is an expert on you or your body except you.

2. Menopause: This is the natural ending of your periods, the average age is fifty-one, but remember women can go through menopause at thirty, forty, fifty, and sixty and are living with it into their seventies and onwards. From the research I have done, you are in menopause after a full year of no periods at all. So looking back, my last period was December 2010, but it took up to approximately May 2011 for the swelling to start, hence the visit to the hospital in July.

So did it take nearly six months for my body to start breaking down under Ms Menopauses relentless bashing?

3. Post menopause: This is considered the time after menopause but by now our bodies are only producing a small amount of estrogen and all our progesterone is gone, so the symptoms will continue. At this time the risk of diseases for women increases due to the low estrogen levels, and as we know, due to not having any progesterone in our bodies. July 2012 was when the relentless bashing from Ms Menopause landed me on my backside where I ended up in hospital and had to stop working, so I reckon all in all it took her a good two years to get me to the point of still breathing but feeling like I was not alive. Don't let her do this to you. Don't let any doctor try and tell you, that she/he knows more about your body than you do. Take the time to find a doctor who listens and is there for you; they are being paid good dollars to look after you, make them earn it. And definitely don't deal with anyone who doesn't show you respect or who doesn't listen to you. With knowledge, Ms Menopause will not be able to affect your life to the degree that she has mine.

We know that menopause can exacerbate existing illnesses or conditions. I worry about my daughter who had childhood asthma and has allergies. I worry about my mate who used to have epilepsy, this only stopped after giving birth, it's all hormonal but with the onset of menopause it could resurface. I worry about a young mate who suffers with migraines, I worry about another woman I know who struggles with a bad back, her physiotherapist has told her it is hormonal. I worry about a young friend dealing with depression, and the list goes on. I worry about that next woman who is out there somewhere who wants to disappear in a puff of smoke.

All existing conditions, regardless of whether they are lying dormant or not, may once again flare up, but will be very exaggerated when Ms Menopause knocks. The truth is that you don't even have to have existing conditions to be affected. You may also deal with conditions or illnesses that you have never had to deal with before in your whole lifetime.

I wish I had the magic pill for you to take to make menopause a walk in the park, who knows, maybe they might have it in the future, just check what is in it first. This chapter has suggestions, tips, foods and what I have learnt, in the hope it will make living with Ms Menopause a lot kinder for you even in a small way. If nothing else, you now have the knowledge and basic education, which will give you, power through your own journey. I am hoping too that the medical community will do the right thing by you all and treat you and your journey with respect and treat all women as valuable members of society.

To summarize, here is the information I have gathered which will help you greatly:

- The first sign can be erratic periods - a blood test can be done to see where you are sitting in menopause. Be aware of this, as by the time I was showing forty-three in that blood test, my debilitating journey had already started. Always get erratic periods checked, it could be the underlying reason for something else happening in your body.
- Blood tests will show the level of where your hormones are sitting. Saliva tests show where your progesterone level is sitting, get this early in your journey and you will have a head start. My test cost $50 in 2013. I think that the saliva test is a more accurate reading.
- Ensure you have pap smears and mammograms every two years. I know, a bit off track, but it's a personal note for the daughter, ok dear?
- Existing conditions or illness can be exacerbated regardless of whether they have been sitting dormant or not. If you do have any

existing condition or illness and if you "see it" or "feel it" even in a very minor way, get it looked at early, it will ease your suffering a hell of a lot by dealing with it in its "infant" stage.

- Ms Menopause can cause problems with other organs, glands, hormones etc throughout the entire body network. I am still gob-smacked and disgusted that the medical community has not alerted us to this. Women who have never had health problems in their life before menopause are all of a sudden dealing with them. Any change in this phase of your life, whether it is physical, mental or emotional, let your doctor know. If the doctor doesn't take it seriously, demand to be listened to, it's your body and mind, you know when something is not right. Listen to your body.

- Another thing I would suggest is making sure you have income protection. For those in the workforce, make sure your superannuation has it. Some do automatically, some don't. Get income protection added on, even if you have to pay a few dollars more. In the long run, if you have to walk from a job or need time off due to Ms Menopause, you will still be able to hold your own throughout it. Also ensure it has disability coverage as well, in case you are out of the workforce long term or forever. You will need doctor and specialist reports, but your body will tell you how you are travelling.

- For those of who work at home caring for your family, look into how you can be covered for domestic duties. If Ms Menopause affects you, it will at times affect the whole household income. Your partner may need to take time off for you. You may need to pay for extra care for your kiddies at times. Being sick is not cheap.

- Enquire whether menopause cover is included. Most likely it won't be but the more of us who inquire about this the more chance there is in the future that menopause will be covered. If you find that it is covered, ask what the conditions are. We all know the battle I had with my insurance company, so always stand your ground with them.

Now I know this all sounds quite drastic, but it's better to be covered for illness, although hopefully you won't need it. You can also organize income protection and insurance on your credit cards. Depending on conditions they can make your payments for you through their insurance if you are unable to work. Look into it, it will be worth it and don't assume it automatically comes with this cover, look into it well.

I personally will not allow any doctor to tell me when I am well again. I will tell them. I will know when I am "back," or even just walking side by side with Ms Menopause and am able to take my rightful place in the world again. Do not let any doctor tell you that you are ok when you know you are struggling, and please do not struggle with Ms Menopause in silence. Those days are coming to an end if I have anything to do with it.

Unfortunately, the sisterhood is not a given when you are dealing with menopause. Some women will support you, others will downplay your suffering. You know your body, don't take it on and don't let anyone make you feel diminished in your suffering or in your search for the answers to the many questions. Remember, at the end of the day you are fighting for you.

Ideally, that bloody medical community will be handing you a cocktail in the future, with an open catalogue of everything you could possibly want to know, and wishing you all the best when Ms Menopause knocks, and thanking you for your contributions, past and future! Oh okay, maybe a fantasy and over the top, but the more women stand up and say, "I am not suffering with menopause in silence, I demand to know the truth," the sooner women will be treated with the respect they rightly deserve in this phase of their lives.

Having to deal with chemotherapy can put a woman into early menopause. Her age will determine her chances of early menopause. A site I read said that the average age for a woman to start menopause is fifty-one, so the closer a woman who is dealing with chemotherapy is to this age, the higher her chances of going into early menopause. They also stated that the percentage gets lower for women who are younger, but sadly it is still happening.

I added this in as going into early menopause is not a commonly known side effect of chemotherapy. Of course always talk to your specialist, but knowing this may help you through your journey.

Menopause-induced depression is very real. Don't let any doctor or anyone in the medical community make you feel that it's just in your head. Hopefully by knowing that it is caused by the loss of oestrogen which affects our serotonin (happy drug) levels you will be more in control of it, or at least be aware of it. You are not alone and it's not just you. If you feel it is getting too big for you, try and talk about it. Or even sob it out to your doctor - you too might score some jellybeans! Or try and talk about it with a loved one.

I am really going to try and put Ms Menopause in the spotlight. In doing so I hope in the future there will be places you can all gather and drink tea or get intoxicated together - wow, imagine that, a gathering of tipsy menopausal women, hooley, sounds like fun! I'm in! Well I will be once I can enjoy a drink again without having to sneak a scotch here and there or having to be careful that I don't have thoughts of suicide. It would be a hoot though if we were all safe, and depending on how many chardys you may have, that would then be a hoosth, hoooth, oops whatever!

A recent TV programme showed how they are organising health centres just for men, like a "men's sheds," so men are able to gather and talk about their health and just meet up to talk. Great idea I thought, so let's do the same and get "women's sheds" organised so we all can gather and hang out.

It is so important you have somewhere to go to chill out and talk to other menopausal women, even for a cry or a laugh. It is also so important that there is a place that your loved ones can go to voice their experiences as well. It is also, I have realised, important that your loved ones get a break as well.

Don't be ashamed of the depression either, it is logical that with the loss of hormones our serotonin levels will be affected. Menopause-induced depression is a coward, it will try and attack you more when you are alone but always be aware of it, as I found out. It can grab you when you least expect it. I assure you, all your loved ones adore you and want and need you around happy and healthy for the rest of your natural life.

Exercise is a great thing to do to increase serotonin levels. Exercise is a natural stimulator of mood hormones including serotonin. Any movements you want to do, or whatever you are capable of, will help, just check that your health is up to it first. For me personally, I'd rather be sitting down with a scotch in hand but for exercise I prefer to walk, it's easy and it costs nothing.

When my mate heard that I had started walking again she thought it was great and this is the sms I sent back to her: "I know. I just got my vitamin D hit, helped to strengthen my bones to stop osteoporosis, made my adrenal glands happy, helped to up my serotonin levels which will help fight the menopause induced depression, hmmm, have I forgotten something? Oh and will help to combat the menopause induced insomnia." So there you go, not only is walking cheap, it helps us menopausal girls in so many other ways as well.

In my life I have exercised, I haven't exercised, I have worked hard for that figure I wanted and I have slothed on my lounge working less hard for that figure I didn't care about. You can't strengthen oestrogen and progesterone like you can muscle. If you have worked hard for that figure you have had all your life, many of you will experience weight gain for no other reason except that Ms Menopause is in your life, but if you start building up the hormones that we are losing, earlier and naturally through foods or even now through BHRT, you may get to keep the figure you have and want.

I need to say something else too. I know I joke about my scotch, oh okay and me chardy, but I really think it is a blessing in disguise that at the moment I am allergic to alcohol. Would I have used it as a crutch through the bad times? Well through the whole feckin visit from Ms Menopause actually! I also know that if I had been drinking to help with the depression it wouldn't have been a good idea. I think with me, it would have added strength to the depression. I know the shrink said it had no bearing on it, but yeahnah.

How do I know this? Well I felt the change after just one scotch when I was at the peak in the menopause-induced depression. My thoughts reminded me of who I am not anymore, not just in regard to enjoying a drink, it was deeper than that, and my thoughts started getting a bit dark again. The depression was taking a pretty good hold, even after just one scotch. It really showed me that the alcohol, for me, wasn't a good idea. Please just consider this if you are dealing with menopause-induced depression.

Wow! The thought just popped up again that I could have been one of those middle-aged women you see on those American daytime shows who, at midday, are still in their silk nightie and high heels, with a full face of makeup and immaculate hair, downing their medication with a glass of vodka! I used to think this was funny, but in reality, yeah, scary!

Before I go on I want to say that although something is natural, it can still be harmful. Different natural products can affect blood pressure, allergies and so on. So as much as I want to do Ms Menopause long term at a reasonable cost, I think a trip to a naturopath could be beneficial. Check it out at your local chemist, you too might get to talk to a naturopath for free. Ms Menopause is affecting parts of your body that you did not even know existed, long before she knocks and you start seeing and feeling signs of her, so keep your doctor informed as well.

A naturopath has reviewed the following foods and recommendations to ensure I am giving you correct and safe information. If I had had knowledge from the start, here is how I would have liked to handle my menopause.

Firstly, when needed I would have started BHRT at the beginning. Why should a natural part of every woman's life be turned into such an exhausting, expensive and debilitating journey when it doesn't have to be like that? I would have wanted to do it cheaply and in conjunction with my everyday life and eating habits. Yes! I would have dealt with Ms Menopause in a very lazy way. Hopefully I will have my life and "me" back down the track and I don't want her ever interrupting my life again. Ms Menopause can come along for the ride, but in the next chapters of my life she will be in the back seat!

I would have started putting more foods in my body that are rich in natural oestrogen and progesterone. These are known as phytoestrogens, which occur naturally in plants and can have similar effects to oestrogen, they are just a little weaker. An eating plan with plenty of the phytoestrogens will do a lot to even out the day-to-day oestrogen level, so that when Ms Menopause shows up there will not be such a big drop in oestrogen.

Foods with phytoestrogens, natural oestrogen are: Flax seed, soy beans, soy nuts, soy milk, multigrain bread, flax bread, alfalfa sprouts, garlic, dried apricots, tofu, pistachios, dried dates, sunflower seeds, onion, almonds, cashews, green beans, blueberries, carrots, watermelon, zucchini, potatoes, brown rice and peanuts.

Foods with both good sources of animal and plant progesterone are: eggs, the yolk is said to be especially good, and dairy products such as milk and cheese. Cow's milk contains high amounts of progesterone. Foods rich in zinc such as shellfish, toasted wheat germ, and peanuts are also good sources.

Foods with phyto progesterone: these help to maintain progesterone-oestrogen balance. A few of these are: yam or wild yam, not those yams also known as sweet potatoes. Vitamin B6 rich foods such as: walnuts, whole grain, soymilk and fortified cereal; these are cereals that are enriched with vitamins and minerals such as iron and calcium etc. Some suggestions are: muesli, all brand, oats and porridge. What? No coco pops or fruit loops? Damn!

Mineral Boron is also beneficial; it seems to increase the body's ability to hold oestrogen. The following are great sources of Mineral Boron that also contain phytoestrogens:

Fruit: plums, prunes, strawberries, tomatoes, apples, pears, grapes, grapefruit, oranges, red raspberries.

Veges: asparagus, cauliflower, beets, broccoli stems, cabbage, carrots, cucumbers, lettuce, onions, soybeans, sweet potatoes, turnips.

As for me, even if I didn't have all my allergies, I ain't a soy or tofu girl, but I included all types of food. Hopefully it will cater for all of your likes. Sorry the lists could not be: chocolate cake and cream, KFC skin, cold pizza for breakfast, lots of white chocolate and for my personal preference, a gawjuz man with a bottle of champagne each day! Oh well, that's life, wait a minute! I should be saying, oh well that's menopause! I have thought though all is good in moderation so hmmm!

Here in Australia, there are two associations you can ring if you need help finding a decent naturopath.

The Natural Herbalists Association of Australia, or

The Australian Natural Therapists Association

I personally believe, natural is the best way to go, the other "synthetic" options are dangerous and horrible, but this is just my opinion. It's your body, the way you deal with Ms Menopause is your choice, and this choice is your right. You also have the right to do your menopause as silently as you want. I chose to do mine loudly as firstly there is nothing subtle about me, but also there is the need to get the education and truth out there into mainstream society. Menopause is a really personal time in our lives and it is hard to talk about most of the ways she affects us, but I reckon Ms Menopause wants us to stay silent and this then allows her to continue to bully the menopausal woman, so that's another reason for me to be as loud as I can be in regard to her.

With fatigued adrenal glands your suffering could be twofold, even threefold. From what I have learnt about healing adrenal fatigue/ exhaustion, it requires quite a holistic approach. Throughout your life, adrenal gland health is one of the major keys to the enjoyment of life, so always try and keep these little suckers happy and healthy.

The time frame to heal adrenal gland fatigue is apparently different depending on what stage they are at:

Six to nine months for minor fatigue

Twelve to eighteen months for moderate fatigue

Up to twenty-four months for severe fatigue

I have even read that it can take up to three years to heal the adrenal glands. Hopefully none of you will have to deal with Addison's disease.

Following are some of the holistic methods to treat fatigued adrenal glands, but maybe they are just great ways to live your life anyway:

Laughing: Yes, I always knew it was good for the soul, now I know it tickles the adrenal glands too.

Exercise: Not heavy duty, moderate is only required. Hey, so while you are walking to help the serotonin levels rise which will help with depression, you are also making the adrenal glands happy.

Do something fun each day: I know, you are most probably thinking, yeah right, who has the time? We all have our own idea of fun and it doesn't have to take a lot of time. Fun can be a small thing that makes your soul happy. It could be playing with the dog, or just chatting to a good mate, so yeah, doing something fun each day doesn't mean you have to plan a big expensive day out for it.

Minimize stress: I know in today's world stress has become just a part of everyday life, but stress should not be to the extent where you are screaming or nearly having an aneurysm over a problem. NB: Don't try and hit the high note in the song "Gloria". The beautiful and talented Laura Branigan who sang it in the 80s, died of an aneurysm. Just sayin'. Try and not stress the small stuff. I have always liked the beginning of this prayer:

> *God grant me the serenity*
> *To accept the things I cannot change*
> *courage to change the things I can*
> *and wisdom to know the difference.*

Surround yourself with people who are positive. Negativity has always annoyed me, sure we all have days when we feel the cup is half empty, but some feel the cup is half empty for all their lives and let you know. I am not saying don't be there for people who need someone to listen to them, but constant negativity can drain you.

So if you can't always be with positive people, always try to find a positive in that person. Be positive yourself, always expect things to work out, always try and turn lemons into lemonade. Don't let a negative person take your positivity away, who knows, your positivity could rub off on them.

Get enough sleep: this will also help the adrenal glands to heal faster. I know at times the following is not possible, but I wanted to add it in. Go to bed no later than 10:30pm. Now I know my twenty-three year old daughter will read this and think, "What the...? We only get started at this time when we go out!" I know at your age it seems impossible, but it will make more sense as you get older and closer to your meeting with Ms Menopause. Apparently the hormonal system cleanses between 11pm and 1am and if you are not asleep at this time, the flushing process will not take place, causing a backing up of toxins. I found this information on a few sites, so there must be something in it.

Breakfast is always important. As I have said to my daughter over the years, it is like putting petrol in the car to get it going. Always take the time to eat a good breakfast. Again, I know in today's world life is busy and bloody demanding at times, but never skip breakfast.

There is a saying, which I have also quoted throughout the years. I found it through my research on adrenal glands. I will modify it for a woman:

Breakfast like a Queen

Lunch like a princess

At dinner eat like a pauper.

Try and make time for a nice, quiet, relaxed breakfast each day before the stresses and demands of everyday life start.

We know that adrenal gland fatigue becomes debilitating with stress and the inadequate production of our hormones. We know now that because our hormones and glands rely on each other, by caring for one part of our body, others parts will also benefit.

The following is from Sarah's website, *The Healthy Home Economist*. These are foods that are good for the adrenal glands:

Vegetables in high amounts of fibre, and high in essential vitamins, minerals, carbohydrates and antioxidants are:

Broccoli, cabbage, sprouts, cauliflower, green and black olives, carrots and spinach. These foods strengthen the immune system, and keep the adrenal glands healthy.

Cherries, kiwi fruit, apples, grapes, papaya, mangoes and oranges are also great, just eat them in small servings.

If you are dealing with adrenal fatigue though, go lightly on fruits especially at breakfast. Avoid figs, dates and raisins. These all have fructose and potassium in high quantities and are not good for the adrenal glands.

Try and have at least 120 ounces of protein at breakfast and lunch, this will help to maintain blood sugar. Meat, fish, chicken, eggs, and dairy products are all good sources of protein. I have always hated weighing food, so I don't really know how much 120 ounces is, but from what I am gathering, it's not much, but you will work it out.

Sara also recommends throwing out white processed salt and replacing it with a sea salt. Salt helps the body to maintain hydration and blood pressure. This in turn will help reduce muscle weakness, increased thirst and lethargy, and regulate heart rate. And always get your blood pressure checked by your doctor.

Replace coffee with green tea…ooooh, yeah can't do this! Avoid coffee as it is a stimulant, and fruit juices as they stress the adrenal glands. Chocolate, excess sugar, fast foods, alcohol, fried foods, aerated drinks and caffeine need to be avoided if you are dealing with adrenal fatigue.

Try to combine fat, complex carbohydrates and protein in every meal and snack; the body will need to be replenished at regular intervals.

Complex carbohydrates are bread, rice, corn, cereal, pasta, carrots and potatoes. Green veges contain less starch and more fibre making them great complex carbohydrates. Some are green beans, broccoli and spinach. Sugar is a simple carbohydrate. The complex carbohydrates take longer to break down in your body than simple ones. They help the body to maintain a steady blood sugar level.

Try also to avoid negative thoughts and anger.

Eat meals with people who make you happy.

Minimize stress, eat healthily and exercise.

Now as I was writing all of this, I could hear my twenty-one year old self saying to me, "Who are you? You would have run from someone giving you this advice when you were me at twenty-one. You would have thought being healthy needed constant full on exercise and a diet of stuff that had no taste and the consistency of cardboard. And as for giving up coffee, you still drink your coffee in heat waves!" So, yes I do know that I never, ever, ever thought I would be the one writing about how to have healthy adrenal glands, or that insulin and gallbladders would amuse me, but as I have always said, we are never too old to learn something new.

Mental note to the universe: Why didn't I get to write that book called "Pigging out on fine foods around the world, chatting to God and shagging Mr Right"? Or even that other book that has "50 shades of the colour in between black and white." Hmmm? I get to do the whole Ms Menopause book? Well you know what Universe, I feel very honoured to be writing about Ms Menopause and I hope it helps women the world over, so I say thank you for this opportunity.

Ok, so to answer my twenty-one year old self I say, "But you always exercised on and off and ate good foods, you just didn't appreciate the health benefits of them, you ate them because you liked them. Yes you lived your life and enjoyed junk food and nice wines as well, so you my twenty-one year old self are really not much different to you at fifty-four years old. The only difference is, except for the obvious thirty-two years, that I now know so much better how our body works and I know how and what foods have certain goodies in them to help our body be healthy and happy in this phase of our life.

"So not much has changed except thirty-two years have passed and you my twenty-one-year-old are now menopausal. Ok, rightio, and you have more wrinkles and grey hairs and bits of you may not be as supple as they once were but trust me you will grow nicely into all your ages. Yes we have so far had to do battle with Ms Menopause, but I'm hoping that once we get this sorted the rest of your fifties will be as you always felt they would be, and that is that they will be the best years of your life."

Would I have changed anything in my youth or my life before Ms Menopause started circling? To be honest, no. I have enjoyed my life, even when hardship and grief were a part of it at times, but looking back I wouldn't change a thing. My lifestyle has not created what I am dealing with now, it is as simple as losing those hormones in menopause. I would perhaps be more aware that an "adrenal rush" comes from the two adrenal glands. Oh and it might be an idea not to tell my twenty-one-year-old self that I now enjoy rice milk, I think that would be too much for her! I used to do coffee with one sugar and milk. I now do coffee less, but with rice milk and no sugar. My twenty-one-year-old self would be happy though to hear that I still can't "do" green tea!

Actually, there is one thing I would change, and it's a personal note to the daughter. I would have started saving a bit more seriously in my younger days. I know you can't put an old head on young shoulders, and youth is there to be enjoyed, but amongst all the fun, believe it or not, you can squeeze away a few dollars each week, which will one day turn into a "cha-ching" amount. Otherwise no, nada, not one thing would I change. I have had a wonderful life I just want to get back to it.

Just one more thing, if your adrenal glands get totally depleted, you have Addison's disease. The change of skin colour and excessive salt cravings are two symptoms of Addison's disease which will lead to a lifetime of daily medication, so once again, keep these two little suckers happy.

Another interesting piece I read was in regard to peppermint. This is the relevant part:

> Peppermint is cooling in summer and also helps relieve the hot flushes of menopause. The menthol in peppermint tricks the nerve endings into believing that the body is up to seven degrees cooler than it actually is.

Cool eh? A suggestion is to have a cool(ish) bath or footbath with twenty drops of peppermint oil in the evening, apparently it will reduce hot flushes and help you snooze the night away. I always wondered what women did for menopause before all the man-made synthetic stuff came along and before men started chopping bits off women.

If we look at all the natural things we have at hand like the sun for vitamin D, the foods I have mentioned which have natural oestrogen and progesterone in them, peppermint to cool the body and help with hot flushes, then I have to think that there is much more out there which I haven't yet learnt about. Oh, yes, it rains so my car gets a wash. I think there are healing things in the world that can and have always been there to cater for our needs.

Phew! Thanks God, I personally believe you are a pretty cool dude, I have never lost my faith through this journey, but it has been really tough at times and one has to wonder why? I was hoping you would come up with the goods for us women and it seems you have.

I also want to say thank you to the naturopath who has a column called "Ask the Naturopath" in our local Sunday paper who stated, "Depression descends on many women during menopause." Thank you, and thank you again for putting it in print. When I read it I said to anyone who would listen and who was at home at the time, "Finally it has been said." This naturopath also went on to say that St John's Wort is the best herbal medicine for this and that The Bach Flower Remedy Walnut also helps. I suggest you check all ingredients and make sure they are suitable and safe for you. I am just overly careful due to my allergies, but even without allergies you don't want to overdose yourself on natural products either.

Collagen: Firstly, Vitamin A cream is good for collagen production, but can make the skin more sensitive to the sun. Foods that are good for putting collagen back into your body are Omega 3 fatty acids, fish oils, flax seed oils, Vitamin D, Vitamin C, dark green veges like spinach, red fruit and veges such as red peppers, beets, tomatoes, blue berries, black berries, salmon, tuna, cashews, almonds, green and black olives, fresh cucumber, fresh stalks of celery, raw carrots, baked sweet potatoes and avocado. Also, did you know that avocado contains the same omega fatty acids as fish? Soy protein, milk, cheese and hummus also are good to help with collagen. Other suggested collagen fix-ups are: Avoid too much sun, have good nutrition, avoid too much stress and ensure you hydrate with drinking water.

Vitamin D: I have looked into three ways of getting this very much-needed vitamin back into your body:

The best way to get your vitamin D intake is the sun. Of course we have to be careful with skin cancer caused by too much sun, but where you live and what season it is will determine how much and when you can get your sun fix safely. If you do it safely you cannot overdose and the level of vitamin D cannot be toxic.

You could take a vitamin D supplement which also has calcium in it, but always check with your doctor or naturopath first. Remember, even though it is natural you can still do harm as too much can be just as harmful as too little and this then can affect other parts of your body. We can't feckin win, can we, but I guess it all makes sense. Our bodies are such finely tuned networks, that to finely tune what we are needing to put back in safely will be worth it in the long run and give us back the balance we need to be healthy and enable us to run amok!

Natural foods with vitamin D are cod liver oil, tuna fish, salmon, mackerel and sardines, egg yolk and raw mushrooms. I have only mentioned a few to give you a head start. You know looking at the above I think I realize now why I had a reaction to the Vitamin D tablets I took in the early stages of this journey. I am allergic to all that I have just mentioned, ah ha!

Calcium: Natural foods with calcium include almonds which are very high, sesame seeds, and eating five dried figs daily gives you 135mg of calcium. No figs though if you are dealing with adrenal fatigue. Also spinach, oranges, broccoli and dried herbs such as: dill, basil, thyme, oregano, poppy seed, mint, parsley and rosemary.

So now we know vitamin D is important itself but also for the absorption of calcium I would suggest that in the early stages of your own journey with Ms Menopause, get a blood test to check your vitamin D level.

Now let's talk about the new hope on the block, BHRT, Bioidentical Hormone Replacement Therapy. This is another option for you. These are natural plant based hormones that are pretty well the closest you will get to the natural hormones in your body. There is the natural yam based progesterone and there are natural oestrogens as well. Do you remember my short trip of three months I had with HRT and how hideous it was? Well the ten days of progesterone I had to add to the synthetic HRT was called Provera, which is a synthetic progesterone as well.

I now know that Provera can have severe side effects including nausea, an increased risk of cancer, fluid retention, abnormal period flow, depression and it can increase the risk of heart disease and stroke. Yep I definitely recognise some of them! Here I was blaming it all on the synthetic oestrogen HRT gel.

In Australia natural progesterone is available as a prescription medicine. Products that have progesterone in them are available only on a doctor's prescription. Research has shown that progesterone absorbs nicely through the skin and is not as effective when swallowed by mouth as the liver can break it down before it can exert an effect on the body.

Side effects apparently are extremely rare with natural progesterone. If you do overdose yourself a bit as I did, you may get headaches and tender boobs but that's it. I say it is still a safer method of hormonal replacement than HRT. It is manufactured from soya beans, wild yams and other plants. Today it is produced for pharmaceutical purposes with the aid of an enzyme (an enzyme acts as a catalyst to bring about a specific biochemical reaction.) You will need to find a doctor who specializes in BHRT to get the correct percentage required for your individual needs and she/he will also advise you on where to apply it. It will take a bit of finetuning but it will be worth it. Also you will need a compounding chemist to mix it for you. As for me, I'm going to see if there is a "patch" that can just be stuck on and forgotten about for a while. Whilst rubbing the cream into my skin is easy, I'm thinking if I am doing that until I am eighty-four, a patch would be better. I told you I want to deal with her in a very lazy way!

Too many women in their later years are living with diabetes, Alzheimer's disease, cancers and more, but I believe a lot of this could be avoided if we were able to take control of Ms Menopause a lot earlier. Don't accept anyone in the medical world telling you that a condition that may pop up in your menopausal years is simply ageing. Many of these conditions may never have had to enter your life if it were not for the secrecy and hidden facts that have been purposely kept from us by the medical world.

You may also at times come across those in the medical world who actually think they are God. Don't let them intimidate you. A truly good doctor who cares about your welfare will listen, be respectful, and at times remind us that they are human and may not always have the answers for us. But at least they will admit it and go on to try and find the answers for you.

If you find need to, give your doctor a copy of the movie *Patch Adams* which stars Robin Williams, and tell them that is what you expect of them. Actually I reckon they should play that movie at Doctor School before they are even let loose to deal with patients.

Also don't be afraid to speak up if you know something is wrong with you. The doctors have the certificates hanging on their walls, but it's your body, you are the expert on you! I have also realised we need to listen to our bodies. Our bodies will tell us if something is missing. For example I was craving spinach although I didn't know why, but I listened to my body and then found out it is good for our adrenal glands. The craving I had for cream, was this to do with my calcium levels? I know these are only minor examples and my adrenal glands are suffering, but again, you are the expert when it comes to your body. Listen to you!

Chapter 50

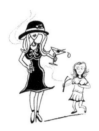

MALE MENOPAUSE IN HONOUR OF ALL THOSE GREAT MEN

This is really being written for my brother but there are many wonderful men out there so let's quickly talk about male menopause.

I was always the first to get annoyed throughout my debilitating experience with Ms Menopause when it was always thrown up that men might go through a form of menopause as well. I am all for everyone having the best and healthiest life that they possibly can, but this was always said in a way which seemed to downplay women's suffering during menopause. From what I have learnt men do have a small amount of oestrogen and progesterone in their bodies, just as we women have a small amount of testosterone in our bodies. I don't know how this affects men but I have learnt that as men get older they lose some of their testosterone and other hormones which can lead to depression, lower energy levels, memory loss and more.

So for all those wonderful men out there, especially my bro, if you are feeling the effects of low energy levels or depression or whatever later on in life don't just put it down to old age. My suggestion would be that you get your testosterone and other hormones in your body checked. It can be rebalanced just like us girls' hormones, naturally and easy. BHRT is there for you guys as well.

Now just a quick word to the Medical World: Why when researching BHRT for men did it always come up as a positive therapy for men and why was it even called an anti-ageing therapy for men, whereas looking into BHRT as a menopausal woman I had to dig deep in the bowls of sites to find it and then had to read about the evils of BHRT for woman and how is not scientifically proven?

Well I will tell you why: Some men, unfortunately, might go through a form of male menopause. All women however, every day, every week, every month, every year, in all generations throughout the entire world will get that knock on their door from Ms Menopause. The profits made from the synthetic and damaging HRT being pushed on women is a sure thing. Hence the positive attitude towards BHRT for men - there is not a more profitable option, and the negative attitude of BHRT for a woman - the profit margins in HRT is through the roof. This however just confirms for me that BHRT works and is a natural and safer therapy for the menopausal woman than HRT. Ok! I rest my case Gov!

Before my journey started with Ms Menopause, I looked forward to it and saw it as a celebration. Going through it I thought, no it's not, humbug! But now I do see that it can be a celebration. Round up Ms Menopause earlier with knowledge, teach her to live with you, not you with her, then go on and have a hoot of a time for the rest of your natural lives!

LIVE WELL... LAUGH OFTEN... LOVE MUCH!

Chapter 51

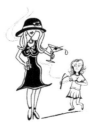

THANK YOUS AND ONE "OH HELLO!"

Thank you to my daughter. I knew from the age of sixteen I was going to have a little girl and she would be known as Bekki. How did I know this? Well yeah, maybe that's another book. My little ray of sunshine came into the world and gave my life purpose. I know this journey of mine has not been easy for you. I started this journey when you were eighteen and you are only now beginning, at twenty-three, to see a glimmer of your real mamma again. I have always been fully aware of how this has affected you, as Ms Menopause also stole from you, but you always knew amidst your busy young adult life, when to give me a kiss or a cuddle, and it was always at the right time. Your timing in making me laugh throughout all of the seriousness and scariness was always impeccable. My struggle to be healthy would never have had been so important if it weren't for you. You are and always will be the core of who I am. Thanks for choosing me to be your mum. And never hide that wonderful sense of humour you have been given.

Always be true to yourself, because you are fabulous enough. We are all human and we all make mistakes. When life seems to take a wrong turn just get yourself back up, dust yourself off and get back into it, oh and shoulders back sweetheart, I am very proud of you. Remember that sometimes when you stand up for things in life that you believe in, you may have to stand alone, but I have every faith in you to know you have and will continue to "do" life well. L'amore sei tu! And remember never underestimate the power of prayer.

Thank you to the best brother in the universe. Not only are you a chef, but not once, whilst getting on with your own life, did you ever make me feel like a burden. You have taken it all in your stride, and just gotten on with it. My journey with Ms Menopause would have been a lot harder and more stressful if you were not here. You truly kept our little family together at a time when I just couldn't. I am sorry you had to hold off buying that new car for yourself throughout all of this but I believe in karma, and all the kindness, care, support and love you have given out will come straight back at you. I admire and appreciate everything you have done for me. I love you long time and am very proud of you. You keep doing the cooking though, you are heaps better at it.

Thank you our wonderful old dog. First and foremost, thank you for not croaking it on Christmas Day 2013, I will always be grateful for that. Yes, this is the pup we brought home in 1998. We will always miss you. You were such a wonderful part of our family and such a great protector of us all. This girl even grabbed a snake and pegged it away from a family member! Even when you were starting to wear down, you would still on occasion gallop towards us like a pup. You saw and heard perfectly when we had your dinner ready. You used your oldness and became deaf and blind when it was time for your medication. You were a resilient old girl, but in this family you had to be, you fitted in very nicely. Thanks for your unconditional love Ginger, our family would not have been complete if you were not a part of it. Back at you with all the unconditional love we have for you too.

Thank you to my work buddy who became my email mate, for being such a wonderful friend. I know that you lost your husband, soul mate, best friend all in one whilst I was dealing with this, and then you had to go on and deal with the grief of losing your mum. I wish I could have been there more for you to help you with your loss and grieving. You always kept in contact and it has always been appreciated.

Thank you to my other friends who have cared enough to try and keep in contact with me or asked someone how I am doing. I never wanted to lose sight of any of you. Hopefully we can all get into the backyard again and have a good gossip – oops, I mean catch up. I miss you.

Thank you to my wonderful doctor. You are the one who has been with me from the start of this journey. You have always been very respectful and always listened. The medical community is very fortunate to have you.

Thank you to the nurses who did my needles. It's not often one can say, "So is it done then, okay ta." You girls do great injections.

Thank you to my BHRT doctor. Where do I start with you? Thank you for having such an interest in women's health and for thinking outside the box. I still want to take you home and ask you zillions of questions. Thank you for always making me feel that I had hope by my side.

Even though we parted company throughout this journey I have always and continue to have great respect for you. Thank you to my lawyer. I know you now have a wonderful office and a wonderful team around you but I remember when, in the early days, it was just you, so the lovely ripple effect still starts with you. Thank you for letting me throw you yet another curve ball. All that you have done, in the three times I have needed your expertise, has been very much appreciated. I owe you a Mars Bar. Oh this curved ball stretched the friendship a bit too much I can nearly hear you thinking?

Thank you to my "Angel Writers". What? You thought I did all this on my own? Yeahnah, I wish I could take all the credit for it. Yes, this is a loopy moment. Thank you "Angel Writers" for your guidance throughout the writing of this book, thank you also for giving me the words and energy when I felt at times I couldn't finish it. Sorry about the swearing at times, but, as we all know, I am human, sometimes a swear word is needed to add strength to an emotion. Thank you again, and I love you all heaps too. Say hi to mum, dad, Helen and Craig for me oh and now also Ginger. I miss them all and am looking forward to seeing them all again, but I ain't ready to see them all just yet.

Thank you to my ghostwriter who came in at the end of my book to tidy it up, prepare it for editing, and turn it into the finished book I have been visualizing sitting on my coffee table. Oh and sorry if I sounded creepy when I said I had been circling you on the Internet for over a year. I know I needed help to get to the end of this book and that is exactly what you did.

Oh, hello Boston! Who would have thought that we would ever welcome a cat in need into our tribe? Who would have ever thought that I would actually ever truly love a cat? Well I didn't, but it has happened. This little girl came into our family after being dumped on a shop counter and after her new owner asked if we could look after her for a "bit" until she got her own life settled in late 2012. I was a bit hesitant at first but I knew my results were showing that my reaction to cats now is very small and she was living mostly downstairs with the daughter in her studio apartment, in the daughter's words though it was her "man cave".

My detachment to this cat soon turned into love and due to circumstances we have officially adopted her. I never knew cats could show love like dogs, I never knew that a cat could whack a bell that has been attached to the bottom of a screen door to let us know she wants in. Yes, we have a cat door but that is on another door. I never knew a cat could play hide and seek and that they love running then sliding across the floor in cat tunnels. I never knew that a cat would want as much love as we do.

I never thought I would love a cat to the extent that I felt my heart break when she was knocked down by a car. There are five other cats around our area but of course it was our cat that this happened to. I guess having a habit of sitting in the middle of the road didn't help, oh dear! Happy to say after much love and care and a gigantic feckin' vet's bill she is now back to being that sociable cat that the neighbours love and that we all adore. Thankfully the old habit of sitting in the middle of the road has gone too! Many a time before the car incident our neighbours and we could be seen getting her off the road. Boston is so much a part of our little tribe now that she knows daytime is outside time and night time is inside time. Who would have thought this little bundle of fur could add so much love to our tribe? And who would have thought I am now nearly ending this book with two subjects I thought I would never talk about: Mr Menopause and a cat? Just goes to show we are never too old to learn something new and we are never too old to love someone new. But I have one last thank you to do.

Thank you to Ms Menopause. Yep! Never thought I would actually be thanking her but I do owe her a thank you. Thank you for opening my eyes to how you really can affect women. Thank you for making me realize that you are a gigantic money making machine and that profit is put before a menopausal woman's health so often. Thank you for opening me up to the fact that there isn't a place or funding for the menopausal woman who is suffering, and thank you again for helping me to realise that there needs to be more medical people who do know how to treat the menopausal woman in a safe and respectful way. My biggest and main thank you to you Ms Menopause, is that you have now made it so that when my daughter's time comes to meet you she will not lose her health, earning power, relationships or sense of self. Because of you, my daughter now will be able to open her door to you with knowledge, education and truth.

I have learnt so much since you knocked on my door five years ago, oh yep and I have suffered so much too, but you have been my biggest life lesson so far in all of my fifty-four years. I started to think a while ago, but am only putting it in print now, that maybe you, Ms Menopause, have always been on the side of the menopausal woman but you too have just been a pawn in the pharmaceutical and medical world's grab for those big fists of dollars. So yeah, thanks, and hopefully you and I can celebrate my health and happiness down the track together, united as it should have been from the very start. Oh my god, does that mean we are starting to bond? Wow! Ok come and sloth on the lounge with me and my new friends, BHRT and Hope. I've got a feeling Ms Menopause that you and I are gonna have lots of fun together in the next chapters of our lives.   ALOHA!

9 780646 949475